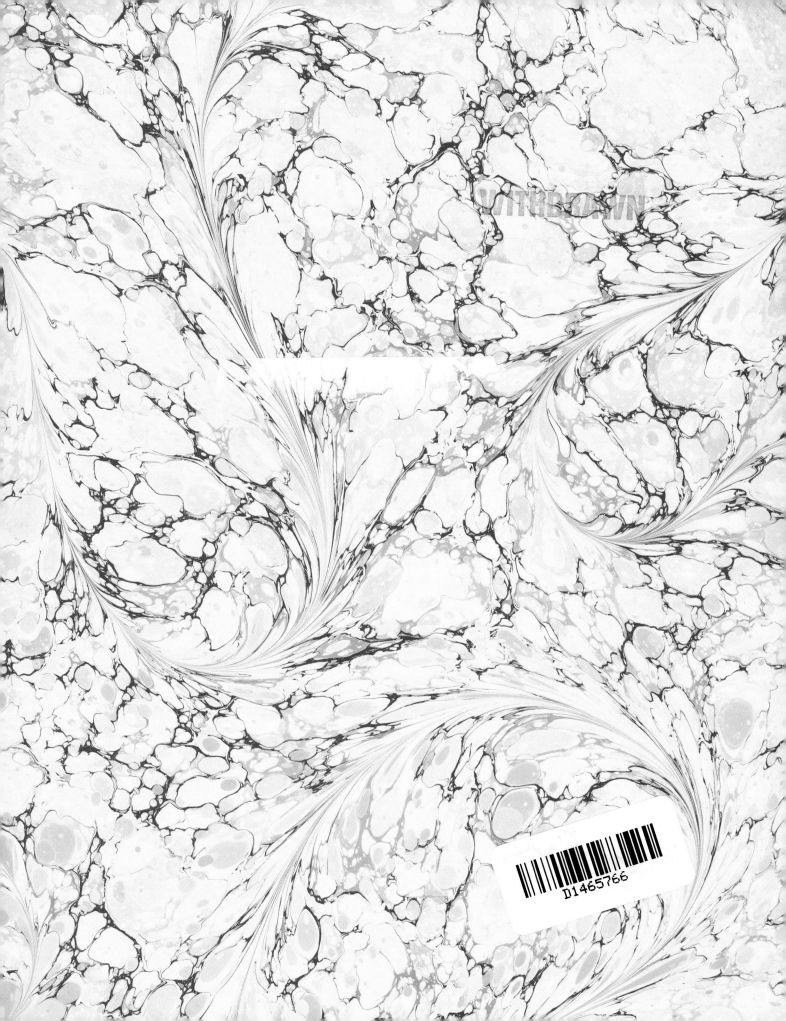

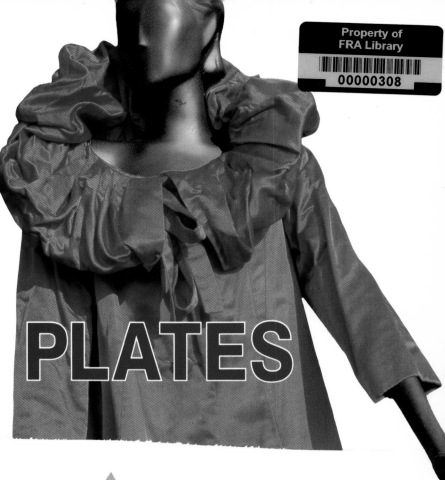

FASHION PLATES

1950-1970

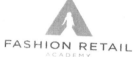
Constance Ko
& Leslie Pi

Schiffer Publishing Ltd

4880 Lower Valley Road, Atglen, PA 19310

Dedicated to the spirit of historic preservation and the
Historic Costume Study Collection at Ursuline College

Library of Congress Catalog Card Number: 97-81351
Copyright © 1998 by Constance Korosec & Leslie Piña

Book design by Leslie Piña
Layout by Blair Loughrey
Typeset in Zapf Humanist BT

ISBN: 0-7643-0438-0
Printed in China
1234

Published by Schiffer Publishing Ltd.
4880 Lower Valley Road
Atglen, PA 19310
Phone: (610) 593-1777; Fax: (610) 593-2002
E-mail: Schifferbk@aol.com
Please write for a free catalog.
This book may be purchased from the publisher.
Please include $3.95 for shipping.

Please try your bookstore first.

We are interested in hearing from authors
with book ideas on related subjects.

Contents

Preface

Fashion Plates 1950-1970 is a look at some typical and some extraordinary costumes worn by both typical and extraordinary women in the fifties and sixties. Some articles are by well-known designers, while others bear no particular name. Whether a designer knock-off or an unrecognized original, some of the unnamed examples are as well-designed and well-constructed as those by the famous houses.

Both authors teach design and/or historic style at Ursuline College, in a suburb of Cleveland, Ohio. Connie Korosec heads the Fashion Department and is an American Studies Ph.D. candidate at Case Western Reserve University (CWRU). Leslie Piña headed the Interior Design Department for many years, and is now Director of the Historic Preservation program. Her Ph.D. is in American Studies at CWRU. Their collaboration is no surprise.

Connie developed and has curated Ursuline's Historic Costume Study Collection since its inception, and, with Ursuline's kind permission, has made it available as the basis for this volume. We would like to thank Ursuline as well as the many generous and thoughtful contributors to the collection — too many names to mention individually. We would, however, like to thank those who lent items from their own collection or inventory: Barbara Johnson Cook, Shirley Friedland, Elaine Doman Johnson, May Brown Korosec, Sandra Burdette Mills, Shelley Stahlman, and Studio Moderne in Cleveland. All items without caption credits are from the Ursuline Collection. Thanks also to Paula Ockner for proofreading.

The photographs were all taken outdoors with mannequins generously given by First Issue, a division of Liz Claiborne in Beachwood, Ohio. Leslie's husband Ramón was the quick change artist who, along with Connie, dressed and undressed, assembled and disassembled, carried and propped the tall, mute, and usually-cooperative ladies, while Leslie searched for just the right scenery and leaned over the camera and tripod. Each photo shoot was dependent on the season and the weather. We tried to represent each season, which we did with considerable success. We also tried to match each costume with the appropriate seasonal landscape, which we did somewhat less successfully. Not always knowingly, we took some liberties and placed winter coats against spring blossoms, or sleeveless sum-

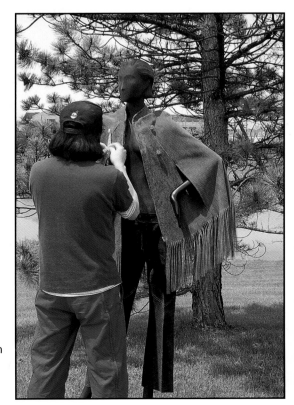

Ramón dressing a mannequin in an early spring landscape.

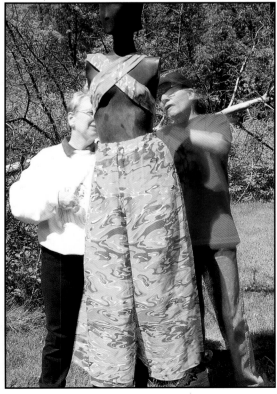

Connie and Ramón improvising in summer.

mer dresses in fall. Sometimes we liked the color combinations, or maybe the item happened to be on the rack. We hope you enjoy the results.

The few snow shots were the most memorable. An especially cold and snowy winter (which is just about any one in Cleveland), plus coordinating three different schedules, made our ideal winter photo session less and less likely. By early spring we knew that we would need to watch the Weather Channel closely and be ready to move if we were to include the required snowfall pictures in the book. One Saturday morning, Ramón and I were packed to go to Tiffin, Ohio to shoot pictures for a Tiffin Glass book. To our surprise and disappointment, when we awoke, it was snowing. Though we knew that the driving would not be fun, we realized that it was also an opportunity, so we scurried to drag a mannequin, a tarp, and a pile of winter coats to the back yard. It was cold and windy, and the snow kept sticking to the camera lens, but we got the winter pictures, which say it all.

All of the pictures speak for themselves, and Connie's knowledge of textiles and fashion should be evident, even without lengthy text. Labels provide information about designer, manufacturer, importer, and/or retailer, and many captions include this data. The timeline can provide the historic context for both those who remember and wore the clothing and for a later generation who can enjoy them equally. As collectible vintage clothing, each article is given an estimated value. This value has little relation to either the original cost or the cost of a comparable new item, because vintage clothing has its own pricing standards. The actual value range for these collectibles is wide, because the sources for purchasing them are so varied. A treasure can be discovered at a thrift shop or a yard sale for a few dollars, while an auction or antique specialty shop in a large city may price good vintage costumes in line with other "antiques." Our value estimates are somewhere in between — they are average retail prices that one might expect to pay for similar vintage items in excellent condition. Of course, *neither the authors nor the publisher can take any responsibility for transactions influenced by our guide.* No guide should be taken too seriously. We do, however, wish you great success and fun in the hunt and in owning, and perhaps wearing, fashion plates like those in the following pages. Seriously.

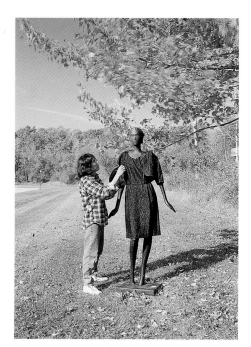

Ramón getting ready for an autumn picture.

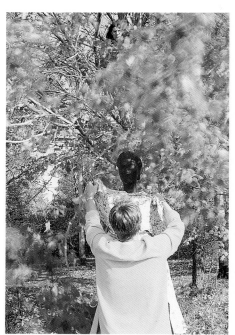
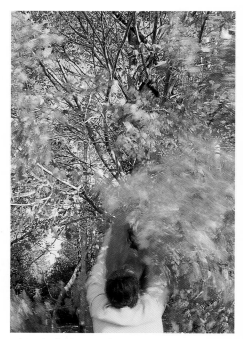

Ramón up in a tree trying to push colorful leaves down behind the mannequin, while Connie struggles to dress it.

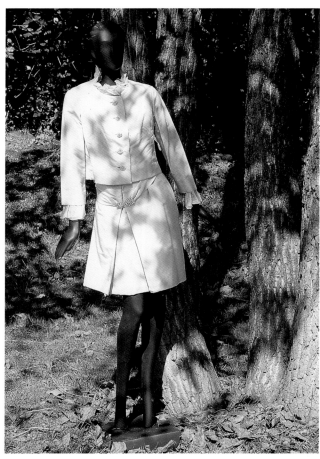

Left: Summer outfit with a shadowy effect.

Below left: Summer costume with a camouflage effect.

Below: Winter coat against spring blossoms with nice color.

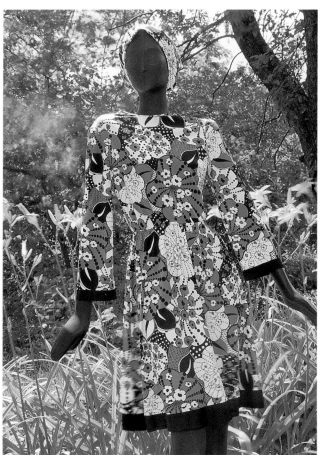

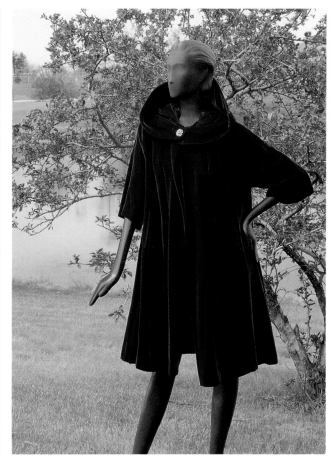

Summer dress against autumn leaves, also with nice color contrast.

Ramón and Connie fixing another summer dress in autumn.

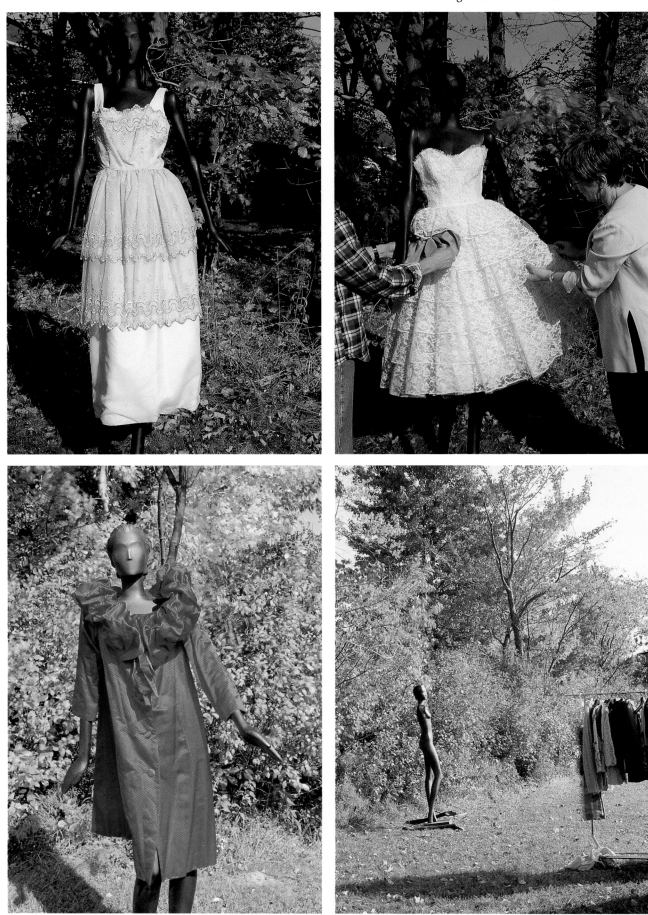

Hot pink coat in colorful autumn setting.

Getting ready with a clothes rack and mannequin.

Fashion in History

1950

Korean War; McCarthy witch hunt begins; U.N. Building in New York; U.S. population 150 million; Ray Bradbury's *The Martian Chronicles*; Margaret Mead's *Social Anthropology*; *Peanuts* comic; contact lenses, Diner's Club first credit card, color television broadcasting; song "If I Knew You Were Coming I'd've Baked a Cake."

born 1950 — Stevie Wonder.

died 1950 — Edgar Rice Burroughs (b. 1875), Al Jolson (b. 1886), Edna St. Vincent Millay (b. 1892), George Orwell (b. 1903), Eliel Saarinen (b. 1873), George Bernard Shaw (b. 1856).

Fashion 1950

Acrylic fibers synthesized.

Pierre Cardin (French) opens in Paris.

Emilio Pucci (Italian) opens his fashion house.

Claire McCardell (American) known for her casual jersey garments and designs for modern career woman.

Christian Dior (French) modifies his "new look" 2-piece suit.

Coats become less full.

Tube swim suit.

1951

Color television broadcasting in U.S.; power steering; Carl Sandburg's Pulitzer Prize for *Complete Poems*; musical *The King and I*; films *African Queen* and *An American in Paris*; songs "Getting to Know You," "Hello, Young Lovers," and "Kisses Sweeter than Wine."

born 1951 — John Candy (d. 1994).

died 1951 — William Randolph Hearst (b. 1863), Sinclair Lewis (b. 1885).

Fashion 1951

James Galanos (American) returns to Los Angeles as ready-to-wear designer.

Pierre Balmain (French) opens his ready-to-wear boutique in New York City.

Shawl collar forms the bodice of a 1950's dress.

1952

Salk polio vaccine, hydrogen bomb; nuclear reactor; Eisenhower elected president with 442 electoral votes; first jet airline service, Sony pocket transistor radio, microwave oven, radio carbon dating; Hemingway's Pulitzer Prize for *The Old Man and the Sea*; John Steinbeck's *East of Eden*; films *Moulin Rouge, High Noon,* and *The Greatest Show on Earth*; songs "I Saw Mommy Kissing Santa Claus," "Your Cheatin' Heart," and "It Takes Two to Tango."

born 1952 — Robin Williams.

died 1952 — John Dewey (b. 1859), Maria Montessori (b. 1870).

Fashion 1952

Hubert de Givenchy (French) opens in Paris.

James Galanos begins to show in New York.

John Cavanagh (Irish) and Victor Stiebel (South African) open salons in London.

Top haute couture designers: Christian Dior, Jacques Fath, Pierre Balmain.

1953

USSR explodes hydrogen bomb; lung cancer attributed to cigarettes; Francis Crick and James Watson discover structure of DNA; Chevrolet Corvette with fiberglass body; fighting ends in Korea; Queen Elizabeth II crowned; Ian Fleming's *Casino Royale* introduces James Bond; John F. Kennedy marries Jacqueline Bouvier; *Playboy* and *TV Guide* magazines; films *From Here to Eternity* and *The Robe*; songs "I Love Paris" and "Doggie In the Window."

died 1953 — John Marin (b. 1870), Eugene O'Neill (b. 1888), Joseph Stalin (b. 1879), Dylan Thomas (b. 1914).

Fashion 1953

Polyester fibers become commercially available.

Mainbocher (American, Main Rousseau Bocher) starts craze for beading evening sweaters.

Giuseppe Mattli (Swiss) creates "Petunia" evening dress.

Bonnie Cashin (American) opens New York salon.

Adele Simpson (American) wins first National Cotton Award.

1954

Nuclear powered submarine *Nautilus;* Ho Chi Minh president of North Vietnam; segregation in public schools ruled unconstitutional; TV dinners; Teflon utensils; J.R.R. Tolkein's *Lord of the Rings,* and William Golding's *Lord of the Flies;* films *On the Waterfront, Rear Window,* and *Three Coins in the Fountain;* Audrey Hepburn wins Oscar for *Roman Holiday;* songs "Mister Sandman" and "Hernando's Hideaway."

died 1954 — Enrico Fermi (b. 1901), Henri Matisse (b. 1869).

Fashion 1954

Coco Chanel reenters the couture industry and introduces tailored, loose jacket with braid binding, plus shirt, blouses, and costume jewelry.

American department stores sell copies of Parisian styles.

Cristobal Balenciaga creates a new "semi-fit" — close to the body in front, easy and straight in back, collars away from neck, soft round shoulders, shorter sleeves — which influences all fashion.

Jacques Fath (French) creates stark color and simple structured shapes; also creates for ready-to-wear market; died that year.

James Galanos produces ready-to-wear with purity of line, flawless workmanship, outstanding imported fabrics.

McMullen cotton blouse.

Indian madras plaids.

Empire-line bolero and sheath dress.

1955

Atomically generated power in U.S.; Peron overthrown; Civil Rights movement begins with bus boycott in Montgomery, Alabama; Disneyland opens in California; Velcro patented; Hovercraft; songs "Rock Around the Clock," "Yellow Rose of Texas," "Davy Crockett," and "Sixteen Tons."

died 1955 — Albert Einstein (b. 1879), Alexander Fleming (b. 1881), Fernand Léger (b. 1881).

Fashion 1955

Anne Fogarty creates "paper doll" look with bouffant crinoline petticoat under shorter full skirts with cinched belts.

Emilio Pucci's vivid and abstract silk jersey prints.

Mary Quant opens London boutique aimed at the under-25 age group.

Herbert Kasper creates couture look for Arnold & Fox at affordable prices.

Coats are tubular and close to the body.

Princess line jacket and A-line skirt 2-piece suit.

Sweater blouses.

"Beatnik" look with black leotard tights, (worn under jumpers by others).

Return of the 2-piece swim suit.

Fad — girls wear man's white shirt with jeans (dungarees).

1956

Transatlantic cable telephone service; Suez Crisis; neutrino produced; Eisenhower re-elected with 457 electoral votes; Grace Kelly marries Prince Rainier of Monaco, Marilyn Monroe marries Arthur Miller; first oral contraceptives used in field test; Rock 'n Roll dancing, FORTRAN is first computer programming language; videotape recorder; films *Ten Commandments; Around the World in 80 Days; The King and I;* songs Elvis Presley "Blue Suede Shoes," "Hound Dog," and "Don't Be Cruel."

born 1956 — Larry Bird, Joe Montana, Martina Navratilova.

died 1956 — Bela Lugosi (b 1882), A.A. Milne (b. 1881), Jackson Pollock (b. 1912)

Fashion 1956

Gustave Tassell opens firm in Los Angeles.

Hardy Amies, top London designer, adopts another Dior creation — the S-line.

John Cavanagh and Giuseppe Mattli are top London designers.

Jacques Heim's three-quarter-length clutch coat.

Victor Stiebel creates fashionable outfits for Ascot and other British horse races.

First major Italian fashion show in New York.

1957

USSR's Sputnik I and II first satellites; European Common Market; Sabin polio vaccine; Eisenhower sends troops to Little Rock, Arkansas; Frisbees; Dr. Seuss' *The Cat in the Hat;* Jack Kerouac's *On the Road;* musical *West Side Story;* films *Bridge on the River Kwai, Twelve Angry Men.*

died 1957 — Humphrey Bogart (b. 1899), Constantin Brancusi (b. 1876), Christian Dior (b. 1905), Oliver Hardy (b. 1892), Joseph McCarthy (b. 1908), Diego Rivera (b. 1886), Arturo Toscanini (b. 1867).

Fashion 1957:

Guy Laroche opens in Paris.

Charles Jourdan opens Paris boutique for footwear.

Christian Dior shows waistline in his collection; dies soon after.

Cristobal Balenciaga introduces the "chemise" dress.

Hubert de Givenchy creates unbelted "sack" dress.

Emilio Pucci adds his signature to printed fabrics and begins a trend.

Wraparound coat with dolman push-up sleeves and fur collars.

1958

Pacemaker; Explorer I; NASA; De Gaulle elected president of France; Chinese take over Tibet and Dalai Lama exiled; Pope John XXIII named; microchip; Pasternak's *Dr. Zhivago;* films *Gigi, Cat on a Hot Tin Roof;* songs "Volare," "Purple People Eater," and "Chipmunk Song."

born 1958 — Madonna, Michael Jackson.

died 1958 — Ronald Colman (b. 1891), Colombian Indian Javier Pereira at age 169 (b. 1789), Tyrone Power (b. 1913).

Fashion 1958

Yves Saint Laurent brings "trapeze line" and the "little girl look" to haute couture after Dior's death in 1957.

Raccoon collar coat.

Car coats introduced.

Flowered jacket/blouse worn with pleated shirts of washable synthetic fiber.

Striped knit tops, white duck pants, white sneakers.

Sweaters worn with tight pants, flat shoes, and poppet beads.

Stretch yarns and Hawaiian prints popular in swimwear.

1959

Fidel Castro overthrows Batista and becomes Cuban premier; Alaska and Hawaii become states; synthetic diamond; Xerox copier; *Lady Chatterley's Lover* banned from the mail; James Michener's *Hawaii;* Ian Fleming's *Goldfinger;* films *Ben Hur, Anatomy of a Murder, La Dolce Vita;* songs "Mack the Knife," "Personality," and "High Hopes."

died 1959 — Cecil B. De Mille (b. 1881), Billie Holiday (b. 1915), Wanda Landowska (b. 1879), George C. Marshall (b. 1880), Paolo Venini (b. 1895), Frank Lloyd Wright (b. 1867).

Fashion 1959

Mary Quant creates suits anticipating the 1960s.

Yves Saint Laurent revives the hobble skirt for House of Dior.

Pauline Trigère introduces double-breasted cape coat with draped collar.

Straight dress with its own jacket, called the "costume."

Sportswear market influences every fashion category — short pleated skirt, boyish blazer/jacket, coordinated sweater-blouse.

Television inspires at-home fashion.

Printed silks.

Dress with Japanese kimono top and wide obi sash.

Cashmere sweaters.

Ankle-length mohair plaid skirts.

Sarong wrap swim suit appears.

Quilted jackets with hoods.

1960

Kennedy elected president with about 100,000 more popular votes than Nixon; FDA approves the first oral contraceptive Enovid; laser; OPEC formed; Cassius Clay (Muhammad Ali) wins light-heavyweight boxing title and Ethiopian Abebe Bikila wins the marathon barefoot at Rome Olympics; Vance Packard's *The Waste Makers;* films *Exodus, Psycho, The Apartment;* songs Paul Anka "Puppy Love," Chubby Checker "The Twist," and Elvis Presley "Are You Lonesome Tonight?"

died 1960 — Albert Camus (b. 1913), Clark Gable (b. 1901), Oscar Hammerstein (b. 1895), Boris Pasternak (b. 1890), Emily Post (b. 1873).

Fashion 1960

Oleg Cassini (Italian) becomes the official couturier to Jacqueline Kennedy, who popularized the 2-piece dress.

Cristobal Balenciaga introduces collarless coat with cropped sleeve and empire waistline.

Norman Norell designs culotte suit.

Status suit — unfitted short jacket and big fancy crochet buttons, peg-skirt, welt seaming.

Tweeds popular — blend smart country into town dressing.

One-piece jumpsuits adopted for driving and flying.

One-piece rubberized suits for scuba diving developed.

Bikini wear at home.

One-piece maillot knit suit with low back for tanning.

Swimwear/beach cover-ups introduced.

Mexican poncho substitutes for sweater.

Tennis dresses with lace hems.

1961

Russia sends first man, Yuri Gagarin, into space; Berlin Wall built; Bay of Pigs, CIA invasion of Cuba fails; Peace Corps; Amnesty International; World Wildlife Fund; Irving Stone's *The Agony and the Ecstasy;* films *West Side Story, The Hustler, Judgment at Nuremberg,* and *Breakfast at Tiffany's;* songs Ray Charles "Hit the Road Jack," Kingston Trio "Where Have All the Flowers Gone?" and Marvelettes "Please Mr. Postman."

died 1961 — Gary Cooper (b. 1901), Dashiell Hammett (b. 1894), Dag Hammarskjöld (b. 1905), Ernest Hemingway (b. 1898), Carl Jung (b. 1875), Eero Saarinen (b. 1910), James Thurber (b. 1894), Max Weber (b. 1881).

Fashion 1961

André Courrèges opens in Paris, becomes leader in the introduction of the mini-skirt and pants suit.

Ticking fabrics found in sportswear.

Coats become shorter.

1962

Cuban Missile Crisis; Pop Art symposium at Museum of Modern Art; Jacqueline Kennedy redecorates the White House; Wal-Mart founded; Tennessee Williams *Night of the Iguana*; films *Cleopatra, Lawrence of Arabia, Manchurian Candidate, Days of Wine and Roses*; songs "Days of Wine and Roses," Ray Charles "I Can't Stop Loving You," Four Seasons "Big Girls Don't Cry," Elvis Presley "Return to Sender," and Bob Dylan "Blowin' in the Wind."

born 1962 — Tom Cruise.

died 1962 — e.e. cummings (b. 1894), William Faulkner (b. 1897), Hermann Hesse (b. 1877), Charles Laughton (b. 1899), Marilyn Monroe (b. 1926), Eleanor Roosevelt (b. 1884).

Fashion 1962

Yves Saint Laurent (chief designer for Christian Dior 1957-58) opens own house in Paris; introduces short coat, inspired by work clothes and sailor's peacoat.

Adolfo Sardina opens firm.

Geoffrey Beene opens own business.

Norman Norell recreates "little black dress" and all-time classic suit with clipped jacket, gored flared skirt, patent leather belt, soft bowed blouse.

Textured sweaters worn with shiny black leather.

Rudi Gernreich creates simple wool tanksuit.

Ernst Engel creates serious scuba swimwear with zipper.

Denim becomes fashion statement — denim pants and blue denim shirt.

Plaid coats.

1963

White House to Kremlin "hot line"; Kennedy assassinated; Günter Grass' *Dog Years*; Pop Art show at Guggenheim Museum; films *The Birds, The Nutty Professor,* and *Hud*; songs Beach Boys "Surfin' U.S.A.," Johnny Cash "Ring of Fire," Kingsmen "Louie Louie," and Peter, Paul, and Mary "Blowin' In the Wind" and "Puff the Magic Dragon."

died 1963 — Georges Braque (b. 1882), Jean Cocteau (b. 1899), Robert Frost (b. 1874), Aldous Huxley (b. 1894), John F. Kennedy (b. 1917), William Carlos Williams (b. 1883)

Fashion 1963

Charles Kleibaker starts his company.

Yves Saint Laurent creates fisherman's smock.

Christian Dior house creates evening chemise.

Oscar de la Renta bubble coat.

André Courrèges shows white wool pantsuit worn with white leather boots.

Pierre Cardin creates "Beatle suits."

Mary Quant starts Ginger Group label.

Emmanuelle Khanh starts youth fashion movement in France, rebels against couture.

African safari shirt appears worn with cords.

Layering becomes fashion trend.

Shirtwaist dress worn with a turtleneck.

Tweed overblouse suit.

Raincoat becomes fashion statement.

Short evening gowns.

1964

Lyndon Johnson elected president; U.S. sends troops to Vietnam; Civil Rights Act; Martin Luther King wins Nobel Prize; Harlem race riot; permanent press clothing; films *A Hard Day's Night, Goldfinger, Zorba the Greek, Beckett, My Fair Lady, Mary Poppins,* and *Dr. Strangelove*; songs Beatles "I Want to Hold Your Hand," "Hard Day's Night," and "I Feel Fine," and Mary Wells "My Guy."

died 1964 — Alexander Archipenko (b. 1887), Herbert Hoover (b. 1874), Douglas MacArthur (b. 1880), Jawaharlal Nehru (b. 1889), Cole Porter (b. 1892).

Fashion 1964

British designer Jean Bates establishes the Jean Varon company.

Vidal Sassoon creates geometric "S-point cut" hairstyle.

André Courrèges creates "space age" collection.

Rudi Gernreich creates "topless" swim suit.

Micia (Italian) creates op art beachwear.

Bonnie Cashin designs sportswear worn for evening.

Cristobal Balenciaga's bubble suit.

Quilted raincoats.

1965

The October 17 Sunday *New York Times* had almost 1,000 pages and weighed 7 1/2 pounds; Op Art; films *Dr. Zhivago, Cat Ballou,* and *The Sound of Music;* songs Beach Boys "California Girls" and "Help Me Rhonda," Beatles "Yesterday" and "Ticket to Ride," the Byrds "Turn! Turn! Turn!" Bob Dylan "Like a Rolling Stone," the Rolling Stones "Get Off of My Cloud" and "Satisfaction," and Sonny and Cher "I Got You Babe."

died 1965 — Bernard Baruch (b. 1870), Clara Bow (b. 1905), Martin Buber (b. 1878), Sir Winston Churchill (b. 1874), Nat "King" Cole (b. 1917), T.S. Eliot (b. 1888), Stan Laurel (b. 1890), Le Corbusier (b. 1887), Somerset Maugham (b. 1874), Edward R. Murrow (b. 1908), Helena Rubenstein (b. 1872), Albert Schweitzer (b. 1875), Adlai Stevenson (b. 1900).

Fashion 1965

McGregor introduces "mod" to U.S. market.

Designer John Weitz opens a boutique for men.

Oscar de la Renta opens his own business.

Yves Saint Laurent creates chemise in bright blocks of color, inspired by Dutch painter, Mondrian.

Paco Rabanne (Spanish) creates the plastic dress.

Betsy Johnson designs, while editor of *Mademoiselle* magazine.

Stan Herman produces appealing fashion at affordable prices.

Miniskirt, followed by the micro-mini.

Skinny rib sweater, U.K. name for tight-fitting ribbed sweater.

1966

Television series *Star Trek, World of Jacques Cousteau;* films *Batman, The Chase, Fahrenheit 451, A Man for All Seasons;* songs "Born Free," "Ballad of the Green Berets," Beach Boys "Good Vibrations," Beatles "We Can Work it Out" and "Eleanor Rigby," Lovin' Spoonful "Did You Ever Have to Make Up Your Mind?" Mamas and Papas "Monday Monday," Young Rascals "Good Lovin'," Simon and Garfunkel "I Am a Rock."

1966-1976 — China: tens of millions of civilians were killed in Mao's Cultural Revolution.

died 1966 — Jean (Hans) Arp (b. 1886), Walt Disney (b. 1901), Alberto Giacometti (b. 1901), Buster Keaton (b. 1895).

Fashion 1966

Ben Zuckerman suit with camel jacket reversed to pin stripe fabric of the blouse, with camel skirt.

Yves Saint Laurent creates smoking jacket for women (haute couture).

Paco Rabanne creates space age leather outfits and metal-link plastic discs.

Pierre Cardin creates space age suit and helmet.

Twiggy emerges as the decade's most famous model.

Film *Tom Jones* inspires ruffled nightshirt.

Fabrics show different textures together.

1967

Six-Day War between Israel and Arab nations; Martin Luther King leads anti-Vietnam War march in New York; race riots in Cleveland, Newark, and Detroit; Muhammad Ali's license to box revoked; films *In the Heat of the Night, Guess Who's Coming for Dinner, Blow-Up, Bonnie and Clyde, The Graduate;* songs The Doors "Light My Fire," Aretha Franklin "Respect," Jefferson Airplane "Somebody to Love" and "White Rabbit," Rolling Stones "Let's Spend the Night Together" and "Ruby Tuesday," Tommy James & the Shondells "I Think We're Alone Now."

died 1967 — Charles Burchfield (b. 1893), Woody Guthrie (b. 1912), Che Guevara (b. 1928), Edward Hopper (b. 1882), Langston Hughes (b. 1902), Robert Kennedy (b. 1925), Vivien Leigh (b. 1913), Henry Luce (b. 1898), Claude Rains (b. 1889), Basil Rathbone (b. 1892), Carl Sandburg (b. 1878), Spencer Tracy (b. 1900).

Fashion 1967

Bonnie Cashin starts the Knittery for hand knits.

Ralph Lauren starts Polo line for men.

Elio Fiorucci (Italian) creates chain of boutiques for younger consumers.

Jean Muir opens in New York as new breed of anti-couture, anti-establishment designer.

Yves Saint Laurent creates Knickerbocker suit.

Film *Dr. Zhivago* inspires the look of Russian blouse, long skirt, and boots.

Pyramid silhouette with large zippers.

Knicker suit worn by younger generation.

Belted sweater dresses.

"Nehru" tunic and sharkskin pants.

African prints popular for dresses.

Nylon caftan beach cover-up introduced.
French resort, St. Tropez, introduces 3-color knit tank dress.
Psychedelic and ethnic fashions appear in designer collections.

1968

Robert Kennedy and Martin Luther King assassinated; Nuclear Non-Proliferation Treaty; Nixon elected president; student riots in Paris; Chicago Democratic Convention riots; air bag developed; Hippie movement with rock music and LSD at height of popularity; use of MSG limited; films *2001: A Space Odyssey, Oliver, Funny Girl, The Odd Couple, Green Berets, The Lion in Winter;* songs Beatles "Hey Jude," Doors "Hello, I Love You," Marvin Gaye "I Heard It Through the Grapevine," Rolling Stones "Jumpin' Jack Flash," Steppenwolf "Born to Be Wild."

died 1968 — Marcel Duchamp (b. 1887), Yuri Gagarin (b. 1934), Helen Keller (b. 1880), Upton Sinclair (b. 1878), John Steinbeck (b. 1902).

Fashion 1968

Anne Klein & Co. opens and shows all-American sportswear look.
Calvin Klein Ltd. opens.
John Anthony designs gaucho suit with full pants.
Jacques Tiffeau, a tailor, adds a cape over jumpsuits.
Cristobal Balenciaga retires.
Yves Saint Laurent creates see-through blouse and safari jacket.
Roy Halston Frowick establishes his own firm, "Halston."
Holly Harp opens boutique on Hollywood's Sunset Strip.
Ruffles appear on chemise dress.
Cut-outs and see-through inserts reveal body.
Evening gowns with see-through midriffs.
Bands of jewels appear.
Mini-coat wrap (styled after the bathrobe).
Pantsuits for women are worn on the street.

1969

Apollo 11, Neil Armstrong first lunar landing; Vietnam War protests across the U.S.; 300,000 stoned spectators at Woodstock Music Festival; Dow at 631; in order to escape from Cuba, Socarras Ramirez flew to Madrid while inside the landing gear of a Boeing 707, surviving eight hours with temperatures as low as -8 degrees F.; Sharon Sites Adams in a 31-foot ketch is first woman to sail across the Pacific alone; films *True Grit, Midnight Cowboy, Easy Rider, Bullitt;* songs Beatles "Get Back," Bob Dylan "Lay Lady Lay," Fifth Dimension "Aquarius," The Archies "Sugar Sugar," Creedence Clearwater Revival "Proud Mary."

died 1969 — Dwight D. Eisenhower (b. 1890), Herman Friedland (b. 1919), Judy Garland (b. 1922), Walter Gropius (b. 1883), Boris Karloff (b. 1887), Jack Kerouac (b. 1926), Ho Chi Minh (b. 1890), Ben Shahn (b. 1898), Robert Taylor (b. 1911).

Fashion 1969

Yves Saint Laurent introduces his pantsuit.
Gypsy dress worn with belts, chains, and costume jewelry.
Maxi and midi hemlines gain ground.

1970

Boeing 747; floppy disc; National Guard shoots and kills four Kent State students at anti-war protest; 448 U.S. colleges and universities close or strike; Congress passes Occupational Safety Act; Nike founded; Environmental Protection Agency (EPA) begins operation; New York City Ballet's 500th performance of "The Nutcracker;" fiction, Richard Bach *Jonathan Livingston Seagull*, James Dickey *Deliverance*, Irwin Shaw *Rich Man Poor Man;* films *Five Easy Pieces, M*A*S*H, Patton, Topaz;* songs Beatles "Let It Be," "The Long and Winding Road," Led Zepelin "Whole Lotta Love," Diana Ross, "Ain't No Mountain High Enough."

died 1970 — Charles de Gaulle (b. 1890), Gypsy Rose Lee (b. 1911), Gamal Abdel Nasser (b. 1918) Mark Rothko (b. 1903), Bertrand Russell (b. 1872), Sukarno (b. 1901).

Fashion 1970

James Galanos creates 2-piece evening pants outfit.
Fox-trimmed coat.

Chapter 1
Dresses

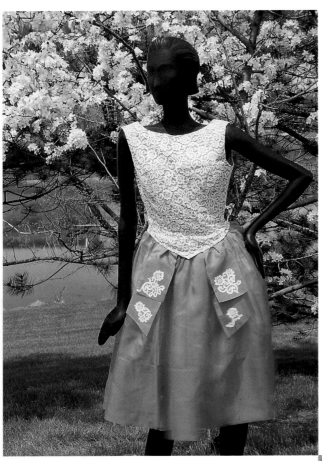

Dress - c. 1959
Light blue 100% silk organza skirt; white 100% cotton lace appliqué bodice, scoop neckline, sleeveless; designed by Shirley Friedland.
$60-$80
Courtesy Shirley Friedland

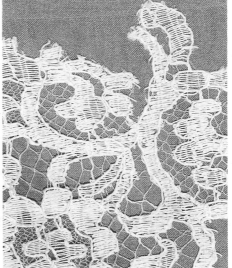

Detail

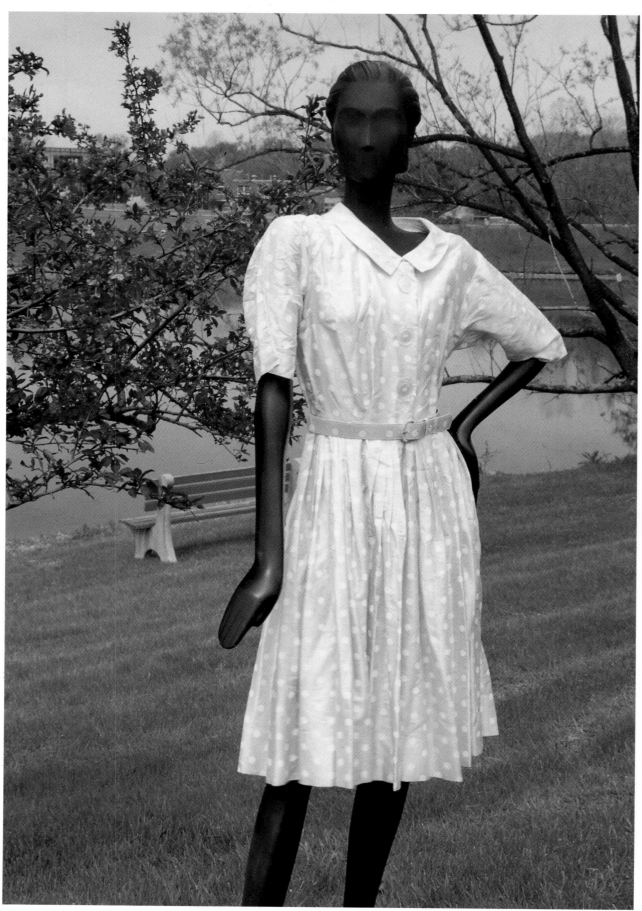

Shirtwaist dress - c. 1950s
Pale pink polka dot 100% silk,
collar, elbow sleeve, belted.
$40-$60

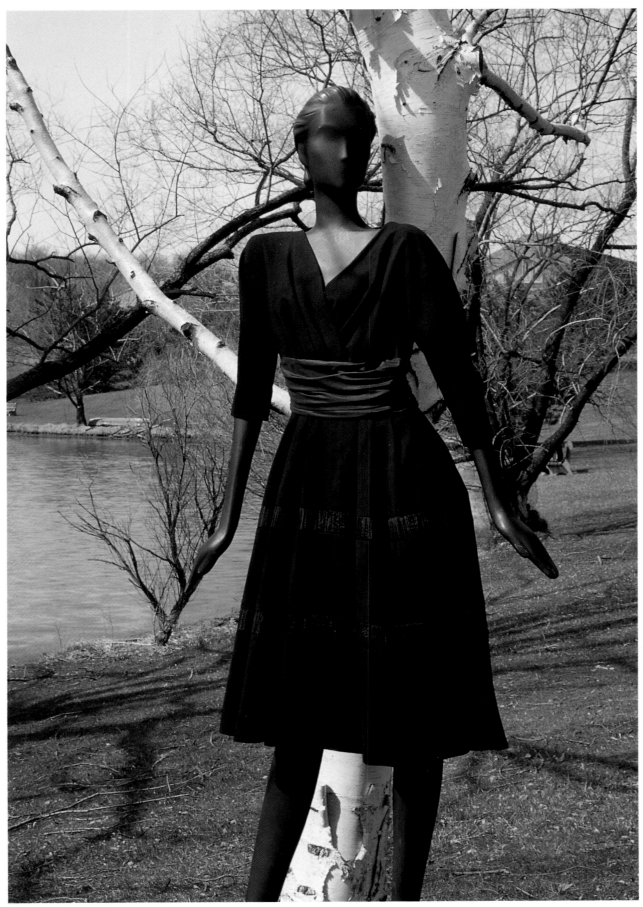

Dress - c. 1950s
Black 100% wool crepe, V-neckline,
3/4 sleeve, cummerbund waistline.
$50-$75

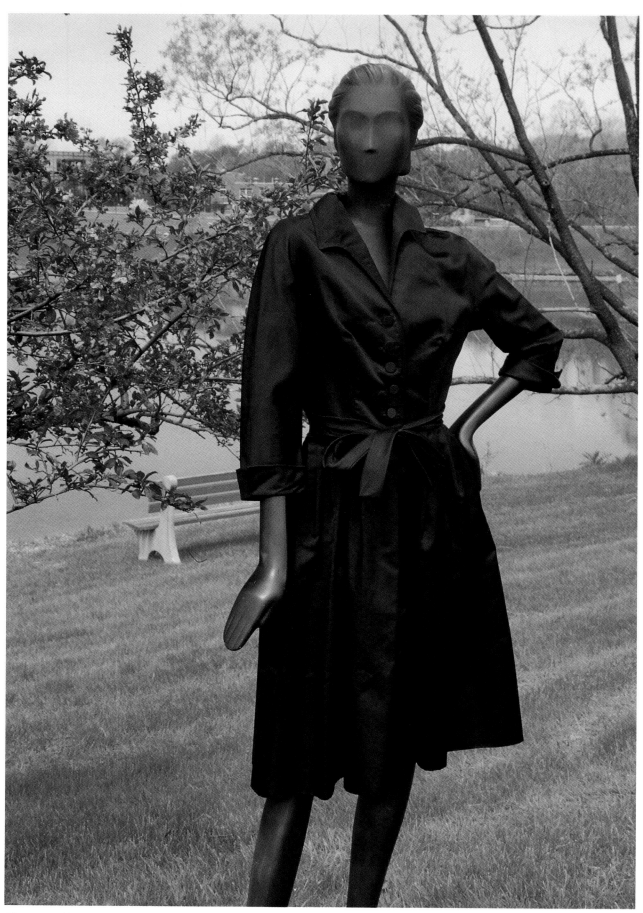

Dress - c. 1950s
Peck & Peck, Fifth Avenue New York
Black satin, curved collar, 3/4 sleeve, belted.
$50-$75

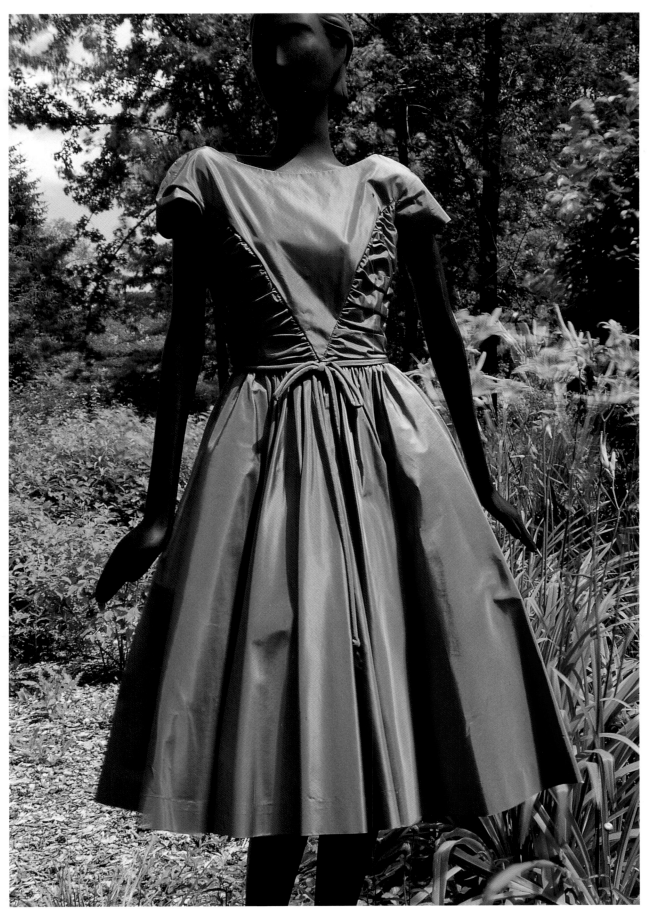

Dress - c. 1958
Blue 100% rayon, cap sleeve, V-bodice,
gathered skirt with tiny bow.
$50-$75

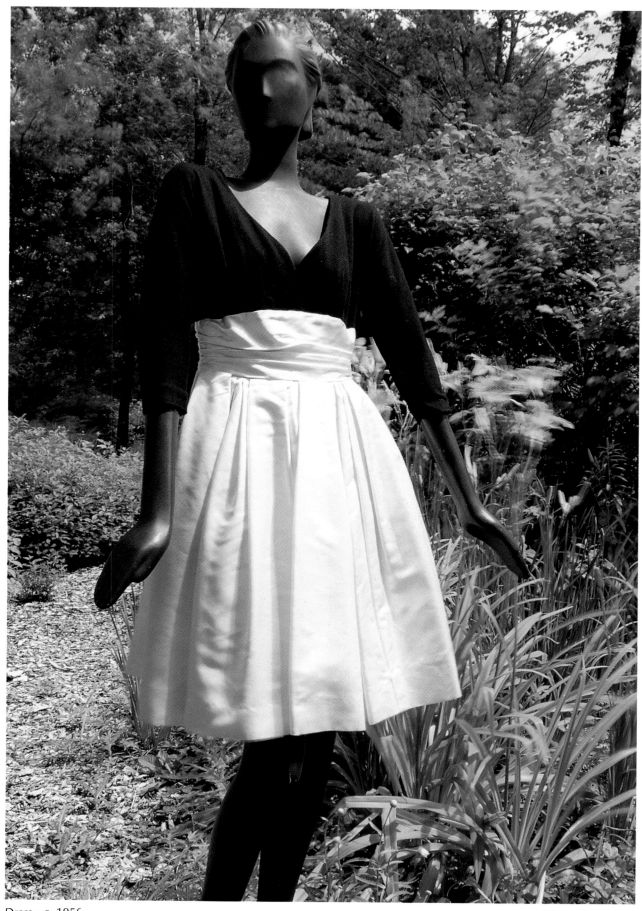

Dress - c. 1956
Melvine Miller, Cleveland, Ohio
Black jersey bodice, empire waistline, 100%
satin box pleat skirt.
$60-$80

Dress - c. 1950s
Yellow 100% linen collar, sleeveless,
patch pocket, embroidery appliqué.
$40-$60

Detail of fabric

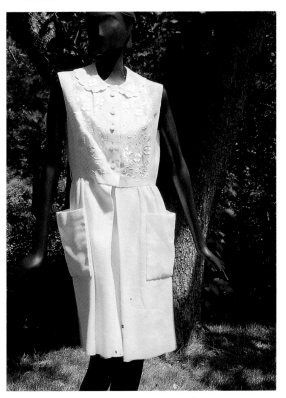

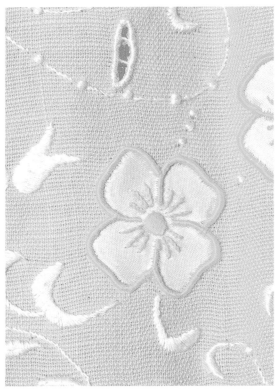

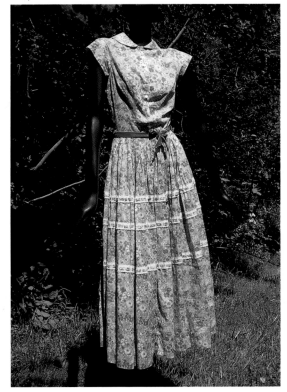

Detail of fabric

Dress - c. 1957
Ethel Joseph, Palm Beach, Florida
Lavender 100% cotton print, collar,
cap sleeve, belted, eyelet trim.
$50-$75

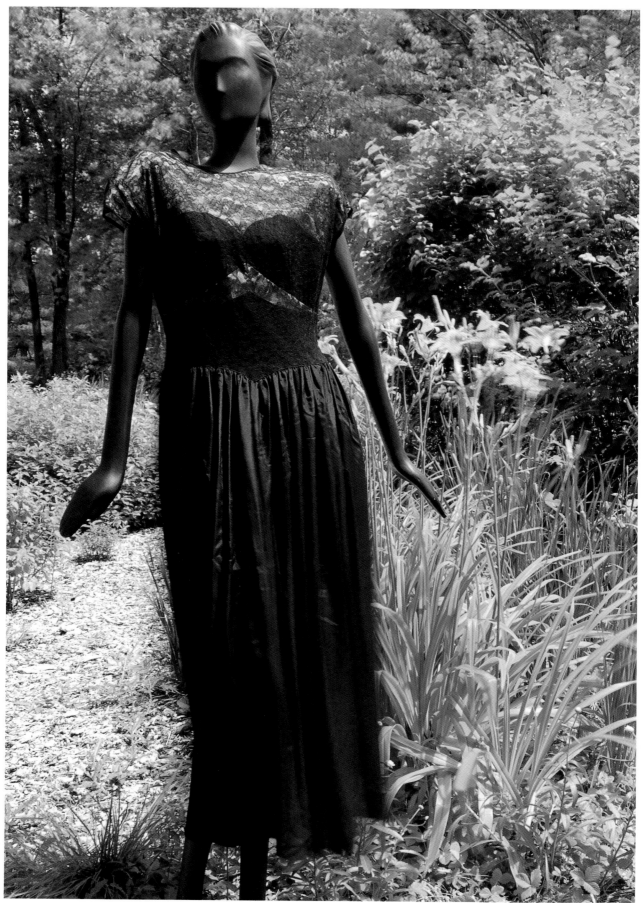

Dress - c. 1950s
Black 100% rayon, lace overlay
bodice, cap sleeve, gathered skirt.
$50-$75

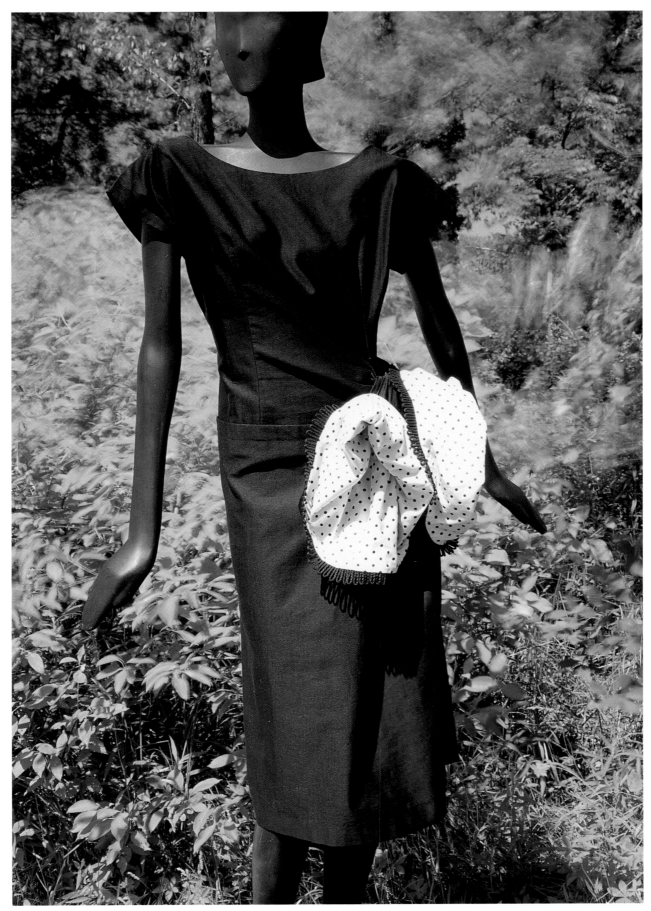

Dress - c. 1950s
Black 100% cotton, scoop
neckline, cap sleeve, drop belted,
white and black polka dot tie.
$60-$80

Dress - c. 1950s
California Girl
Blue 100% nylon print, ruffle collar, long
sleeve, elastic waistline, rope tassel belt.
$40-$60

Detail of fabric

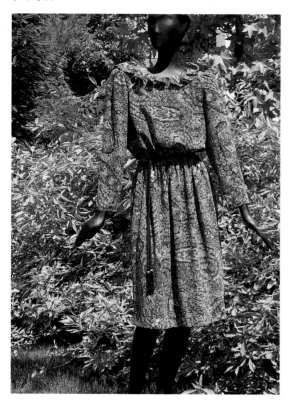

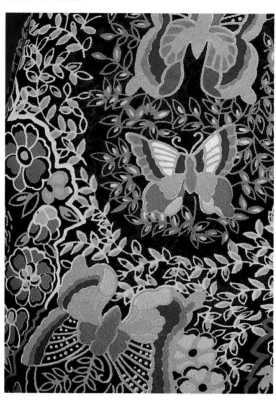

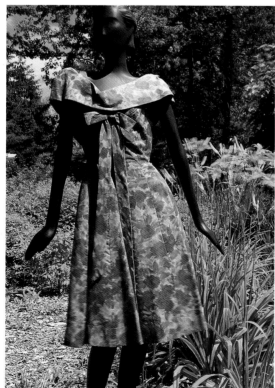

Dress - c. 1958
Gigi Young, New York
Purple 100% nylon print, cowl collar,
sleeveless, bow tie, flared skirt.
$40-$60

Dress - c. 1959
Tanner of North Carolina
Yellow 100% linen scoop
neckline, cap sleeve, belted.
$40-$60

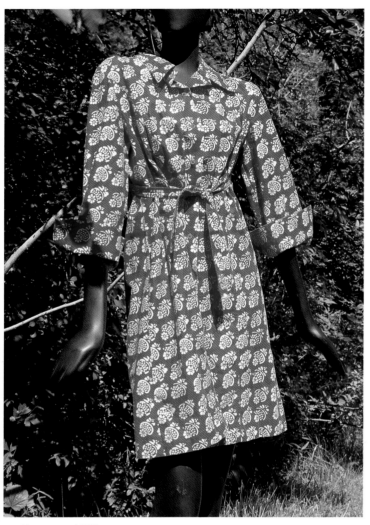

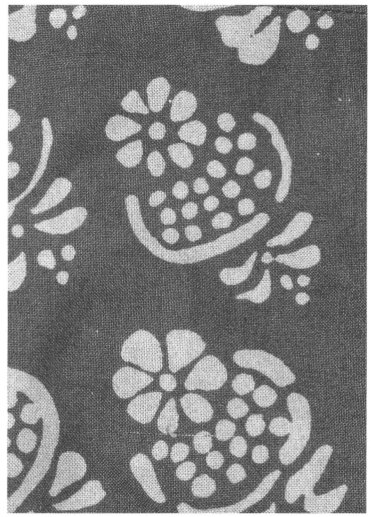

Dress - c. 1959
Marimekko of Finland
Rose 100% cotton print, collar, 3/4
sleeve, belted gathered skirt.
$75-$95

Detail of fabric

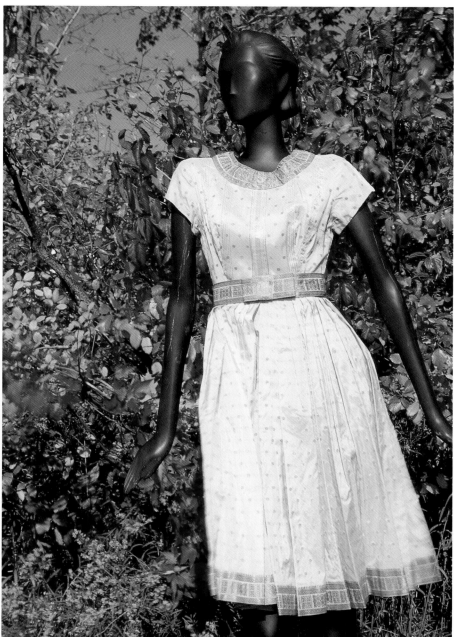

Above:
Dress - c. 1959
Aqua and metallic gold dots, 100%
silk, scoop neckline, cap sleeve,
belted with matching shawl.
$75-$125

Left:
Dress with matching shawl.

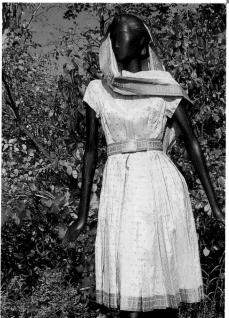

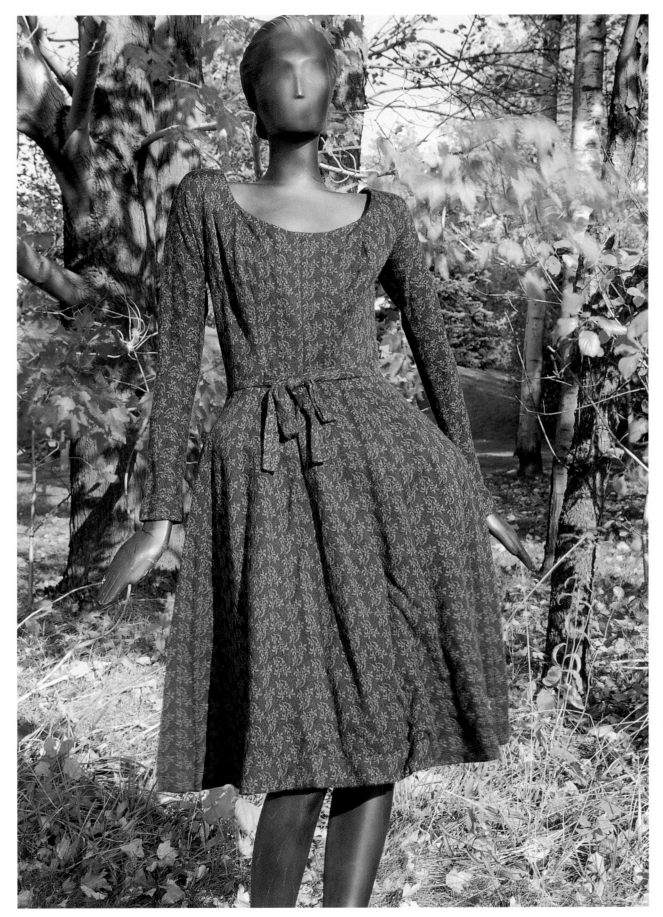

Dress - c. 1950s
Bonwit Teller
Black and purple jersey knit, scoop neckline,
long sleeve, front bow and full skirt.
$60-$80

Dress - c. 1950s
Black 100% nylon, scoop
neckline, sleeveless, full skirt.
$50-$75

Dress - c. 1950s
Carlye
Baby blue 100% cotton, square neckline,
cap sleeve, cording at waistline.
$40-$60

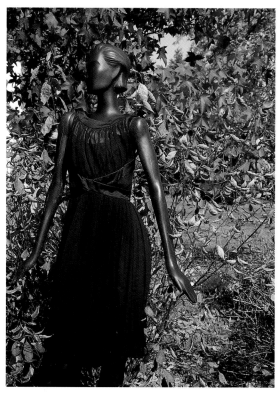

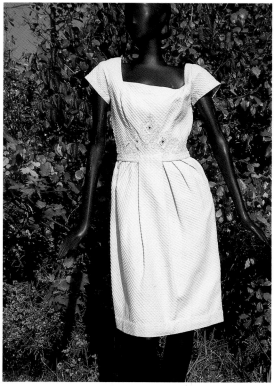

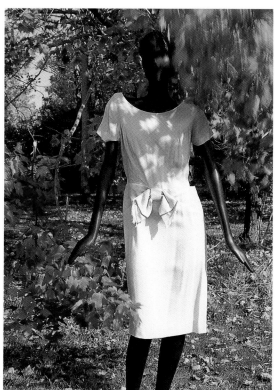

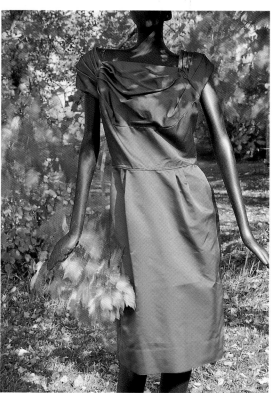

Dress - c. 1950s
Beige 100% linen, scoop
neckline and belted bow.
$50-$75

Dress - c. 1950s
Emerald green satin, square
neckline and cap sleeve.
$75-$95

Dress - c. 1950s
Beige and green 100% linen, scoop
neckline, cap sleeve, midriff appliqué.
$50-$75

Dress - c. 1950s
Navy 100% polyester, Op
Art collar and cuff.
$50-$75
Courtesy Studio Moderne

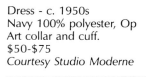

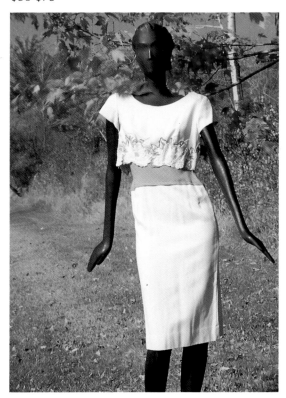

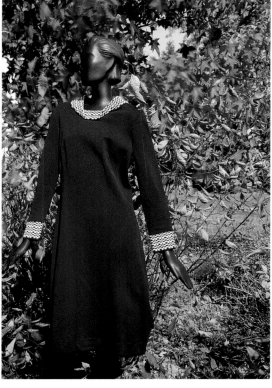

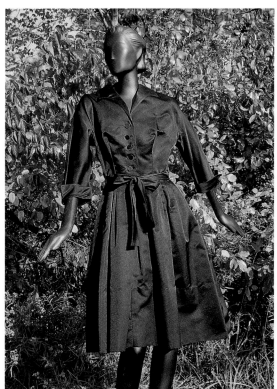

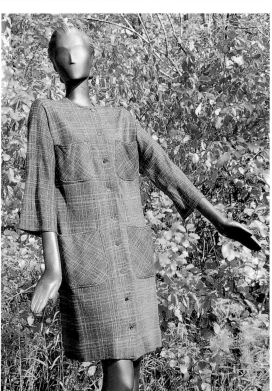

Dress - c. 1950s
Black satin, collar, V-neckline, 3/4
sleeve, cuff, belted gathered skirt.
$50-$75

Dress - c. 1950s
Claire McCardell Clothes by Townley
Green 100% wool plaid, round neckline,
trumpet sleeve, button front, patch pocket.
$50-$75

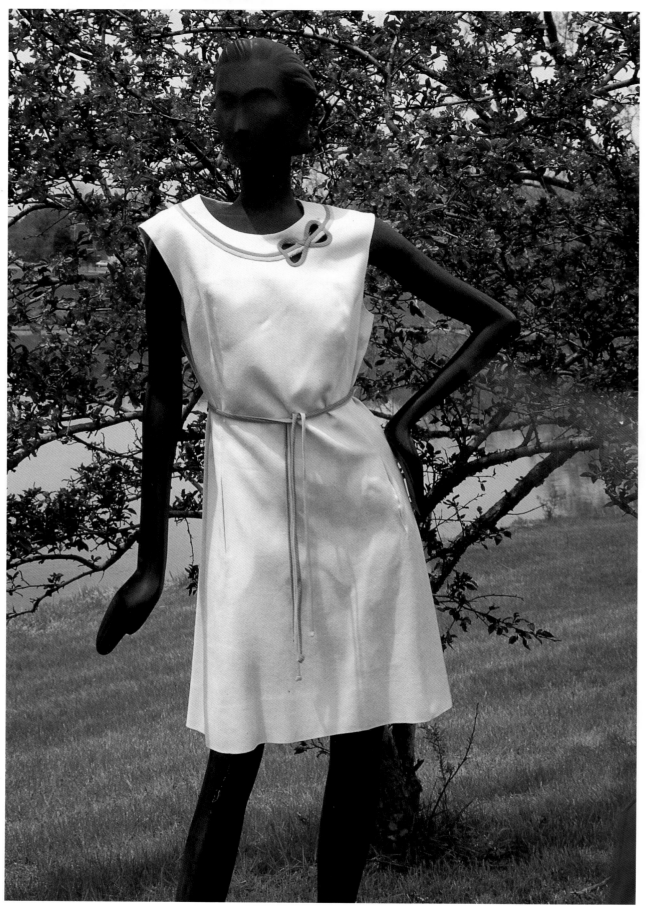

Dress - c. 1960s
New York House of Lords Original
Pale pink 100% linen sheath, appliqué bow
in aqua and hot pink; spaghetti tie belt.
$50-$75

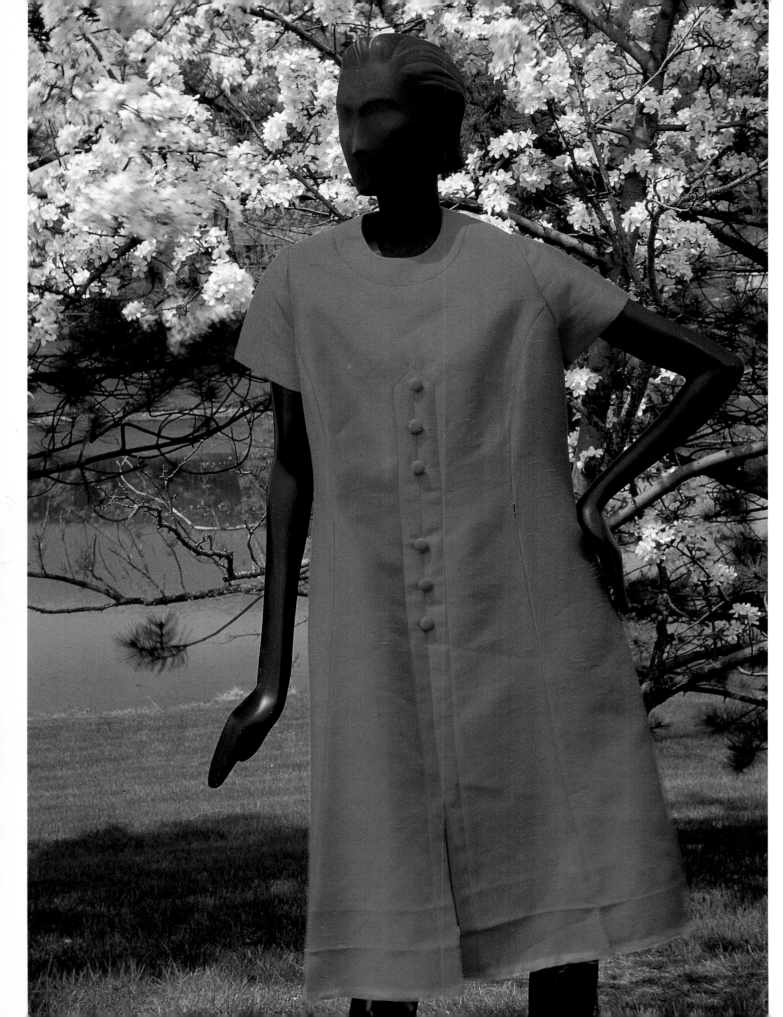

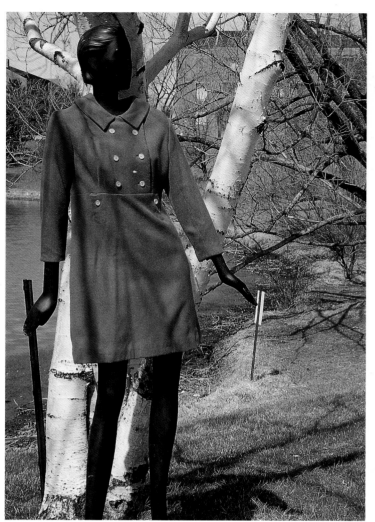

Dress - c. 1960s
Blue 100% wool, double breasted,
long sleeve, slim dress.
$50-$75

Opposite:
Dress - c. 1960s
Rona, New York, Designed
by Patrick Porter
Hot pink 100% silk, round
neckline and cap sleeve.
$60-$80

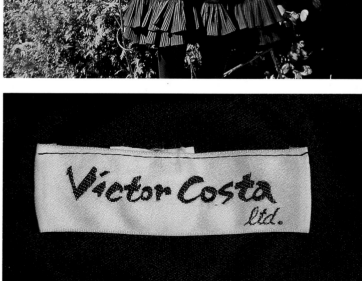

Top:
Dress - c. 1969
Victor Costa Ltd.
Black 100% polyester knit,
ruffled cuff and hemline.
$100-$150

Bottom:
Label

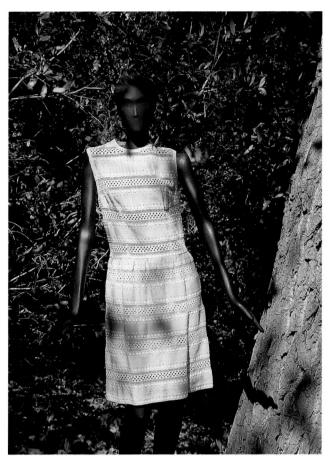

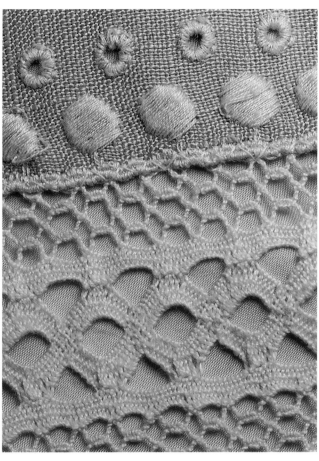

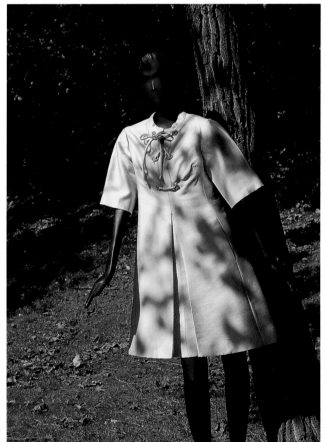

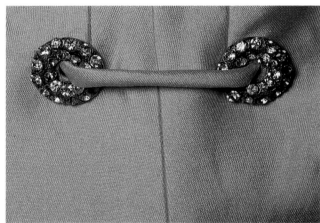

Upper left:
Dress - c. 1969
Pale blue and peach 100% linen, round
neckline, sleeveless sheath, crochet lace inserts.
$50-$75

Upper right:
Detail of fabric

Left:
Dress - c. 1960s
Elinor Simmons for Malcolm Starr
Pink 100% silk, rhinestone eyelet laced bodice.
$100-$150

Lower right:
Detail of rhinestone eyelet

Dress - c. 1969
Brown 100% nylon lace bodice,
cuff, accordion pleat fabric.
$40-$60

Dress - c. 1965
Yellow Swiss dot 100% nylon, scoop neckline,
belted, long accordion pleat sleeve.
$50-$75

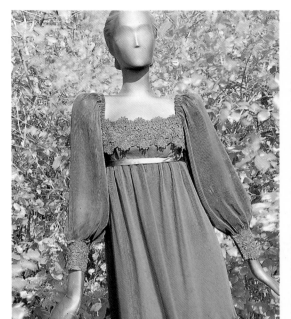

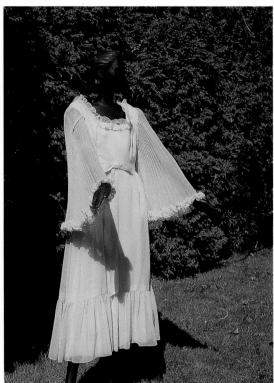

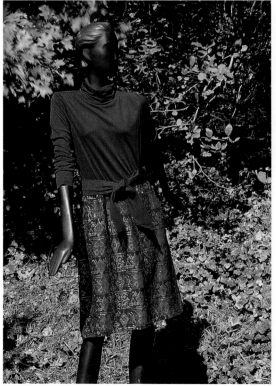

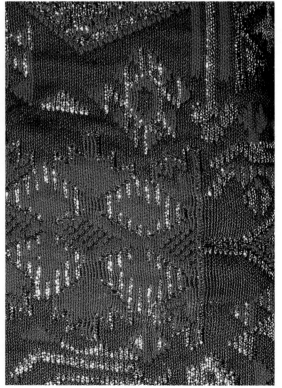

Dress - c. 1960s
Saks Fifth Avenue
Navy metallic 100% polyester knit,
turtleneck, belted geometric motif skirt.
$50-$75

Detail of fabric

Dress - c. 1960s
Red 100% cotton square neckline,
cap sleeve, red geometric motif skirt.
$60-$80

Detail of fabric

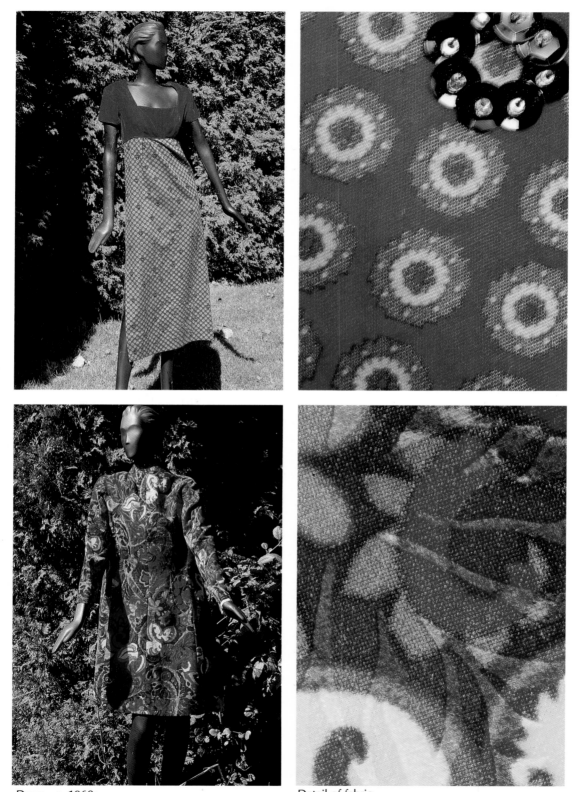

Dress - c. 1960s
Multi-color 100% cotton velour,
round neckline and long sleeve.
$50-$75

Detail of fabric

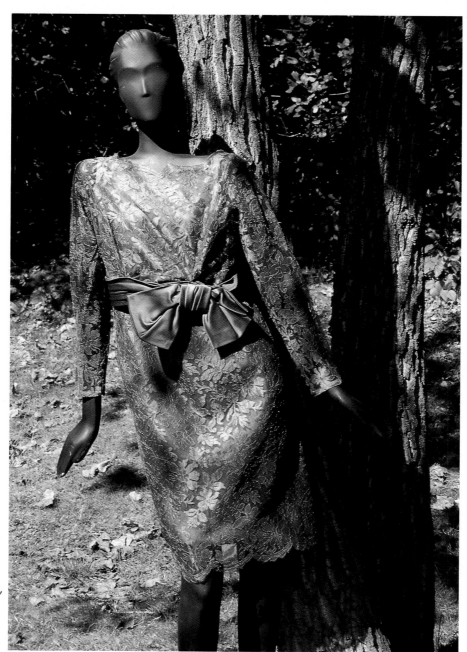

Dress - c. 1960s
Toast 100% nylon, lace,
scallop neckline, long
sleeve, cummerbund
and bow at waistline.
$50-$75

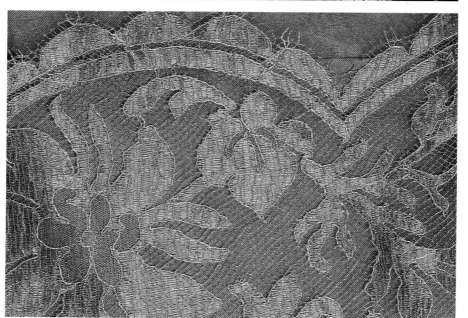

Detail of fabric

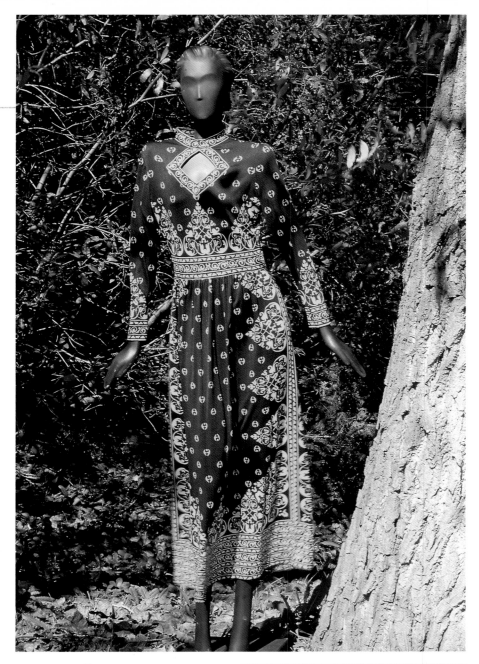

Above:
Dress - c. 1960s
Maurice
Black print 100% polyester knit, banded collar, keyhole bodice, long sleeve, long skirt.
$80-$100

Right:
Detail of fabric

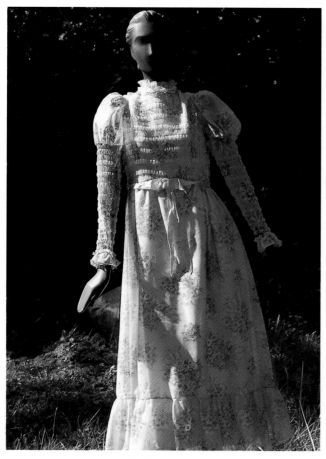

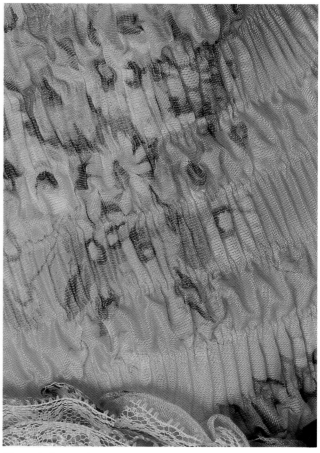

Above left:
Dress - c. 1960s
Pink floral 100% nylon, ruffle
neckline, collar, hem; smocked
bodice and belted.
$60-$80

Above right:
Detail of fabric

Left:
Dress - c. 1960s
Lorrie Deb, San Francisco
Aqua Swiss dot, 100% cotton,
ruffle neckline, cuff, hem; ruffle
dress panels, belted.
$50-$75

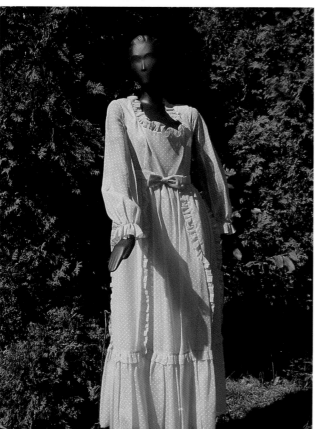

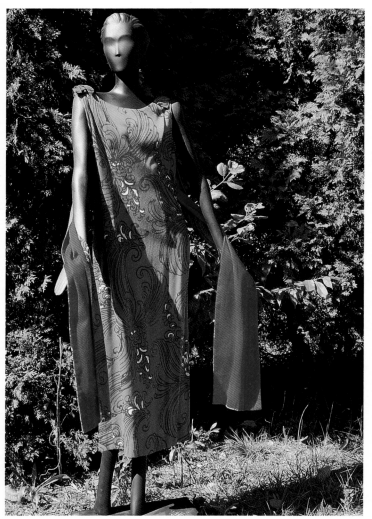

Dress - c. 1960s
Hawaiian Fashions (Sears)
Green magenta print, 100%
polyester knit, scoop neckline,
bows on shoulder, panel back.
$50-$75

Detail of fabric

Opposite:
Jumpsuit - c. 1960s
Jodie, for Halle Bros. Co.
Mock leopard print: 68%
cotton, 32% rayon.
$80-$120
Courtesy Studio Moderne

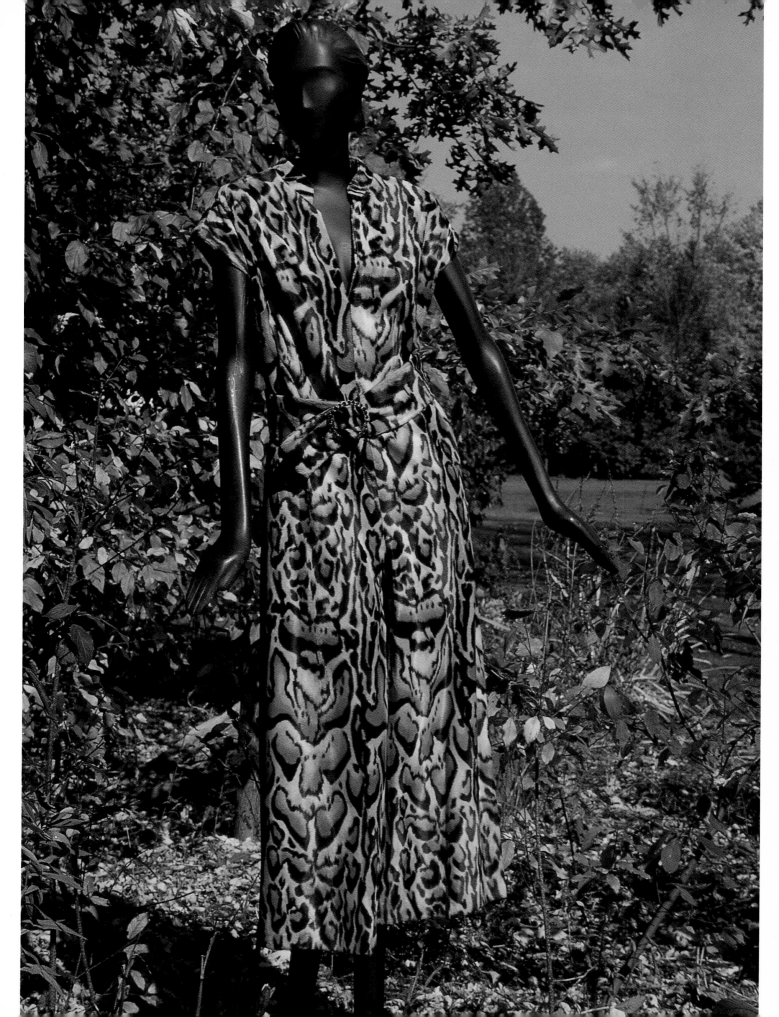

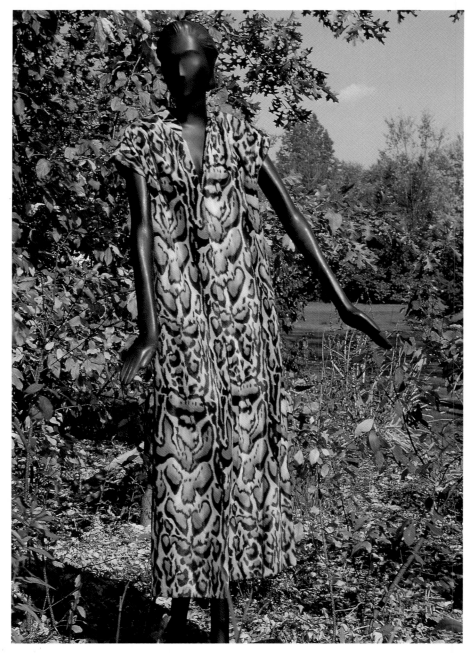

Jumpsuit unbelted

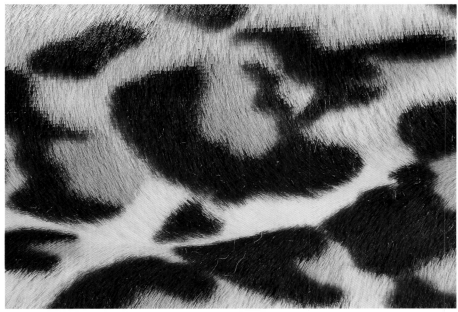

Detail of fabric

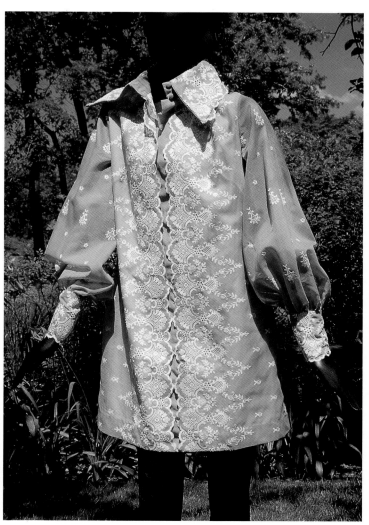

Dress - c. 1960s
Emil, Acapulco
Lime 100% cotton, large collar, bishop
sleeve, cuff, embroidery appliqué.
$60-$80

Detail of fabric

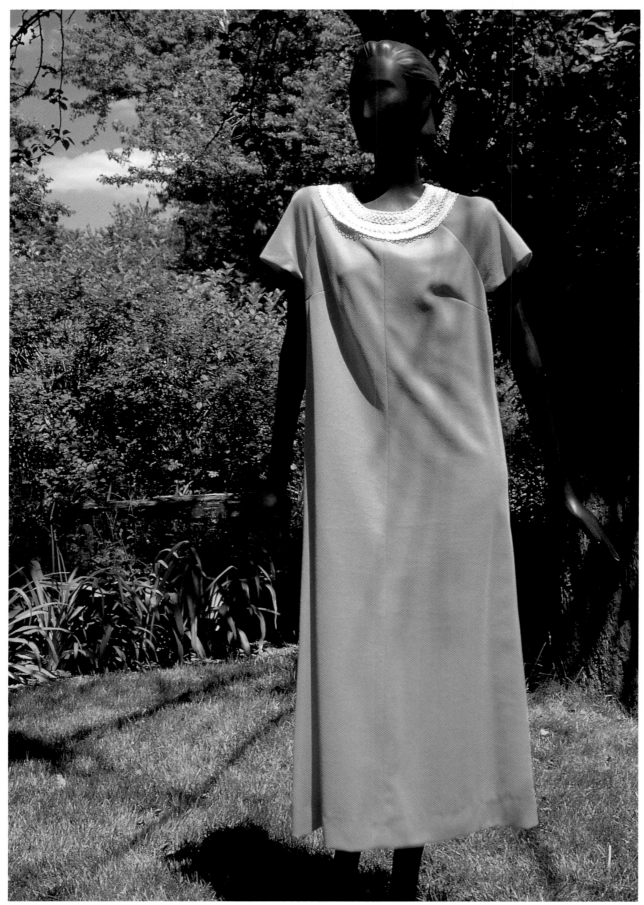

Dress - c. 1960s
Pink 100% polyester knit, silver
braid neckline, short sleeve.
$50-$75

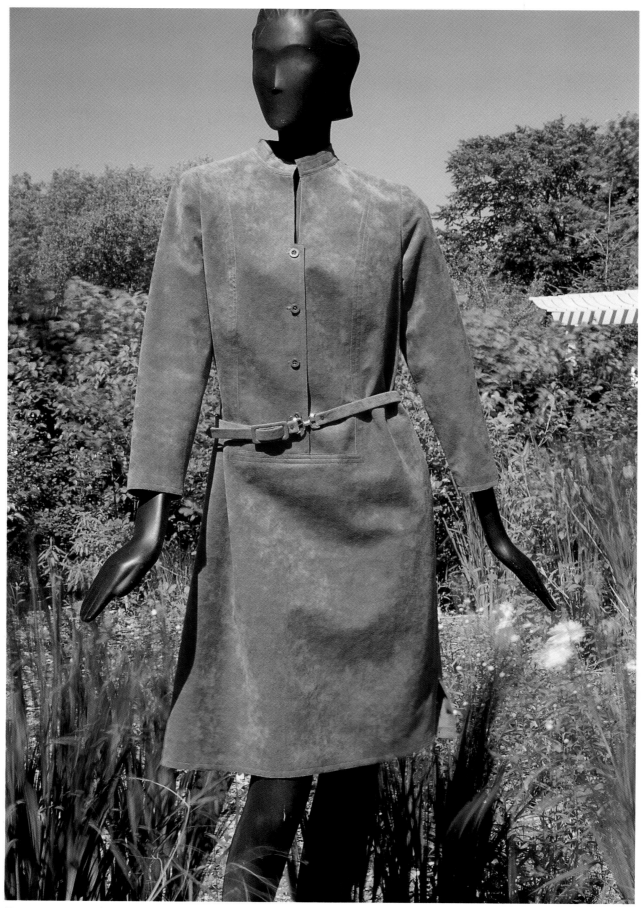

Dress - c. 1960s
Skinner Ultra Suede
Blue ultra suede, round
neckline, long sleeve, belted.
$100-$150

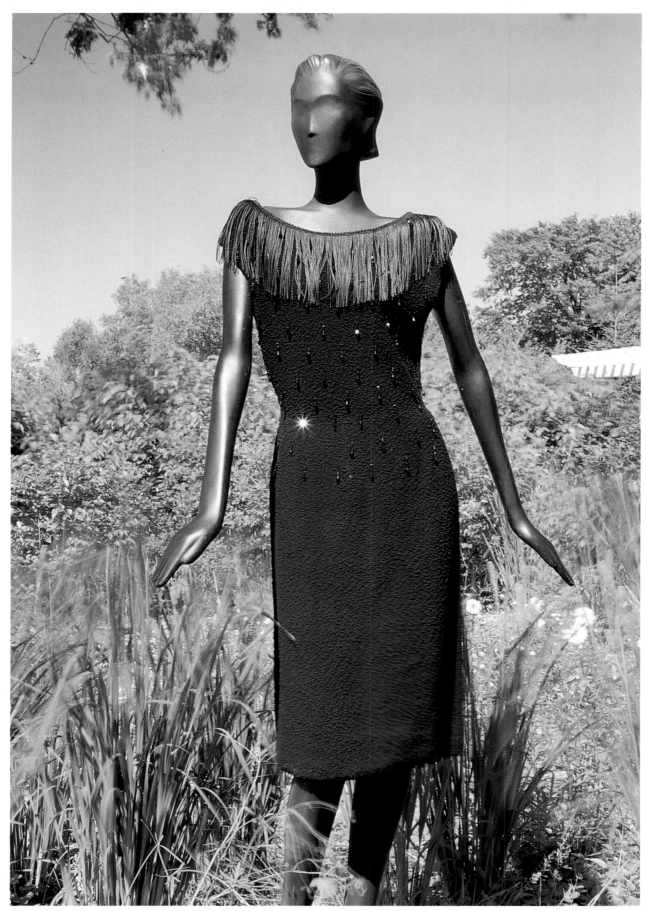

Dress - c. 1960s
Loomed by Hand, Kimberly
Black 100% wool, scoop neckline with fringe, cap sleeve,
tiny teardrop jet black beads on bodice and waistline.
$70-$90

44

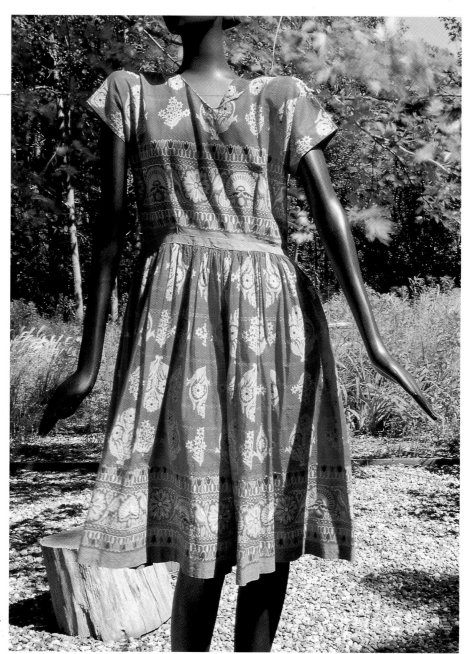

Dress - c. 1960s
Red 100% cotton
print, scoop neckline,
cap sleeve, belted.
$60-$80

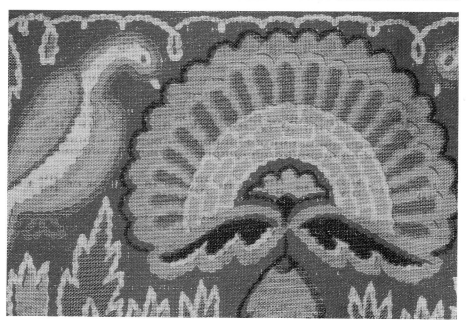

Detail of fabric

45

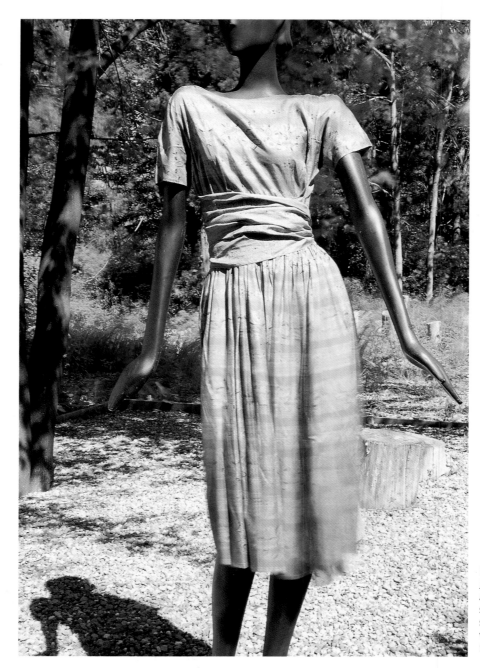

Dress - c. 1960s
Jeanne d'Arc
Aqua 100% silk print,
scoop neckline, cap
sleeve, cummerbund
waistline, gathered skirt.
$60-$80

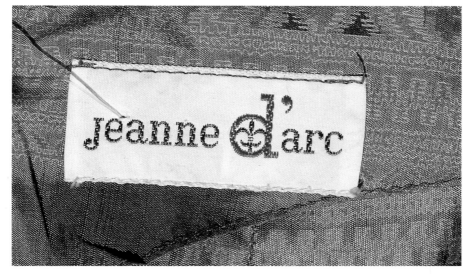

Label

46

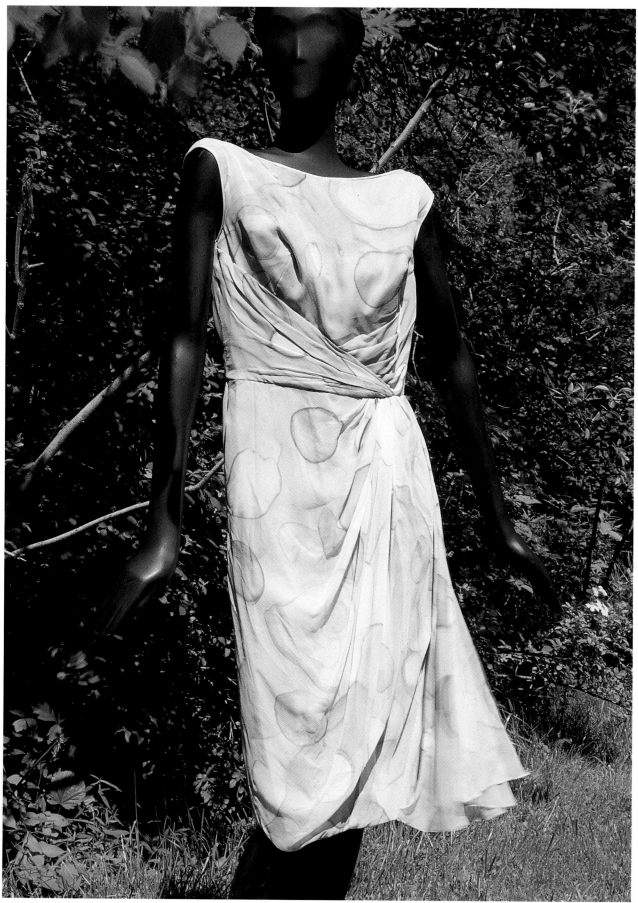

Dress - c. 1960s
Pale blue chiffon print, scoop
neckline, sleeveless, sarong
drape bodice and waistline.
$50-$75

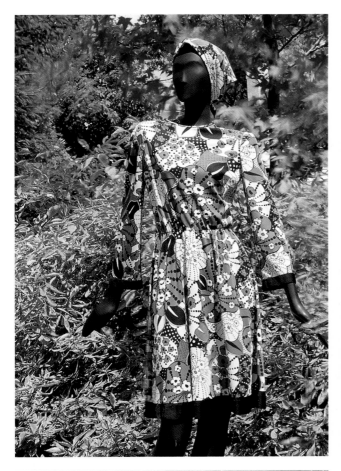

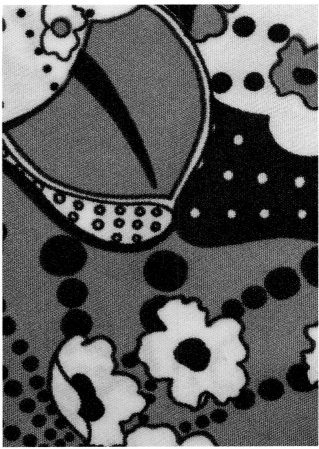

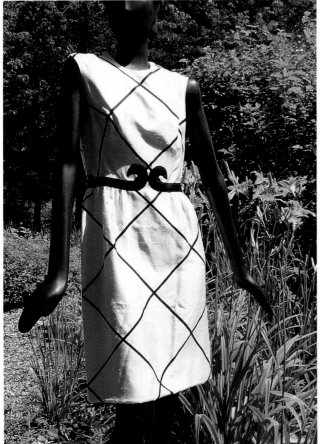

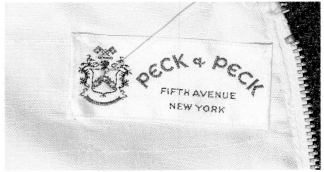

Top Left:
Dress - c. 1960s
Green 100% polyester print, long sleeve,
elastic waistline, triangle head wrap.
$50-$75

Top right:
Detail of fabric

Left:
Dress - c. 1960s
Peck & Peck, Fifth Avenue New York
Cream 100% silk sheath, round neckline,
sleeveless.
$60-$80

Bottom right:
Label

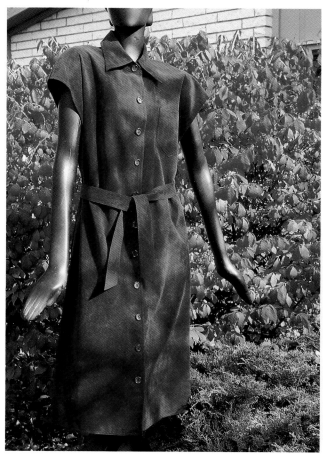

Left:
Dress/jumper - c. 1960s
Blassport
Wine ultra suede, collar,
cap sleeve, belted.
$75-$100
Courtesy Shirley Friedland

Below:
Label

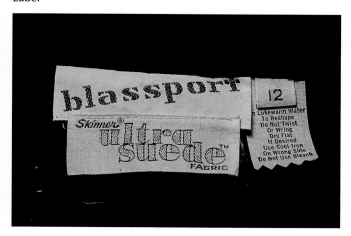

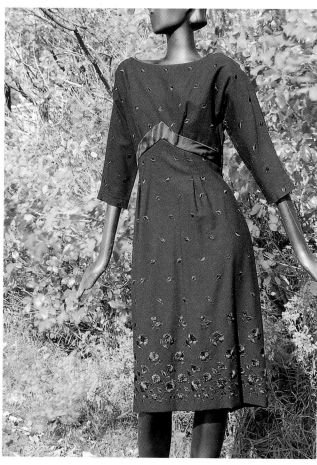

Dress - c. 1960s
Black 100% wool, scoop neckline,
3/4 sleeve, and embroidery motif.
$60-$80

Dress - c. 1960s
Montego Original
Black 100% rayon, scoop neckline, cap
sleeve, black velvet leaf motif at neckline.
$50-$75

Dress - c. 1960s
Black 100% rayon, fitted bodice,
sheer sleeve, straight skirt.
$50-$75

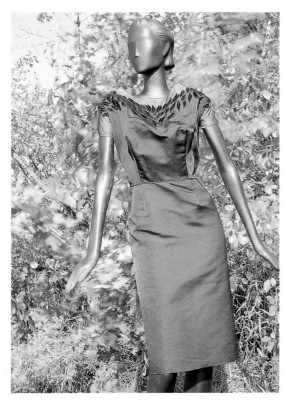

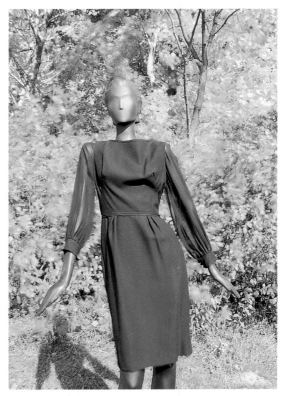

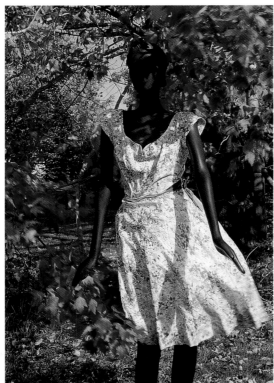

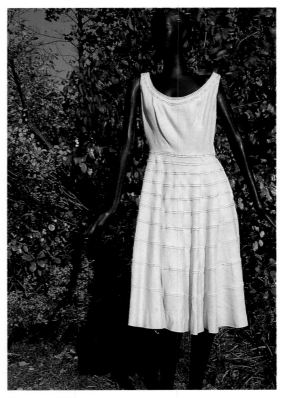

Dress - c. 1950s
Floral 100% cotton, scoop
neckline, cap sleeve, belted.
$40-$60

Dress - c. 1960s
Therese Original by Ted Herman
Pale pink 100% linen, scoop neckline,
sleeveless, belted, rhinestone trim.
$50-$75

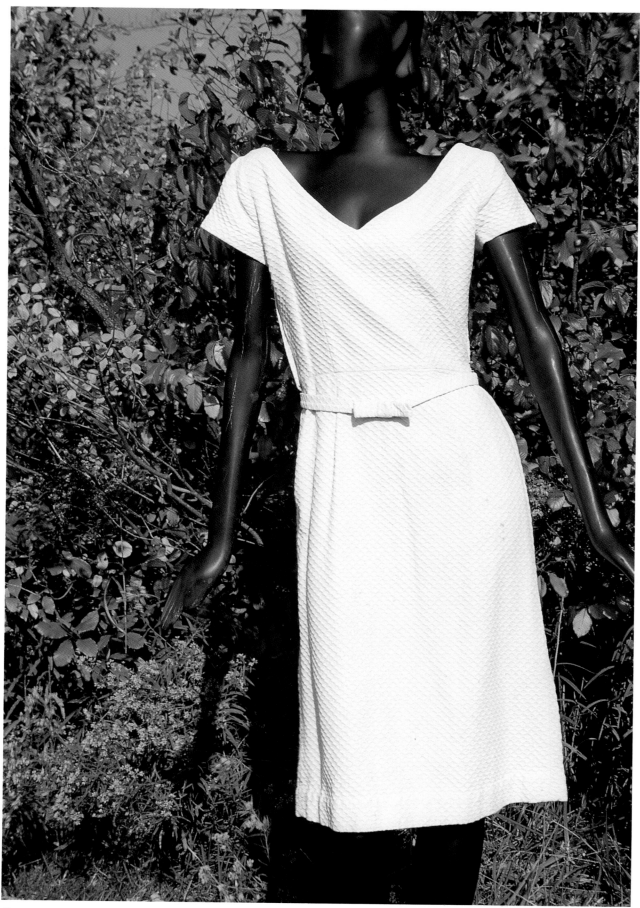

Dress - c. 1960s
White cotton waffle
piqué, belted sheath
$50-$75

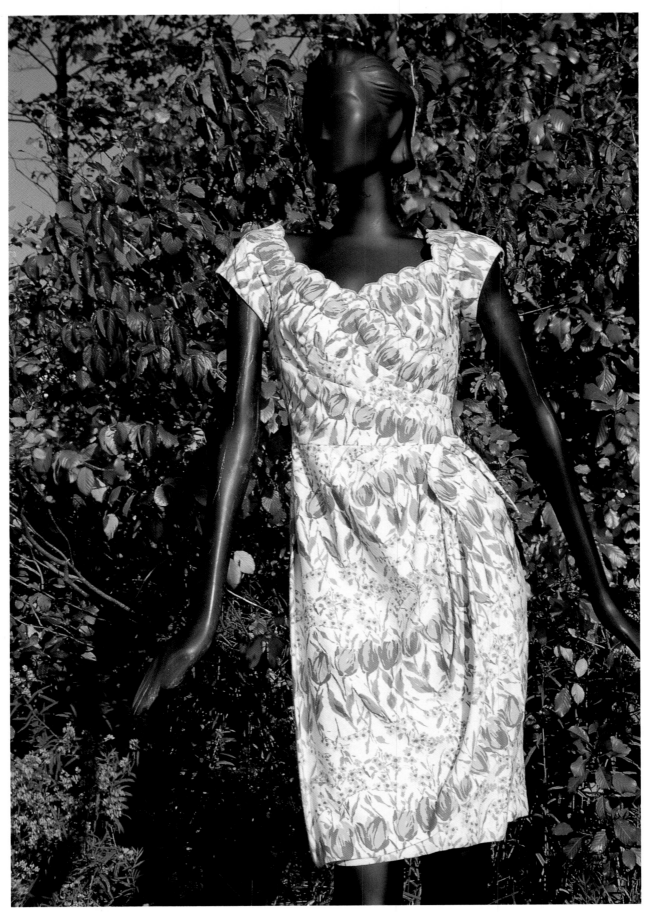

Dress - c. 1960s
Floral 100% cotton
sarong wrap dress.
$50-$75

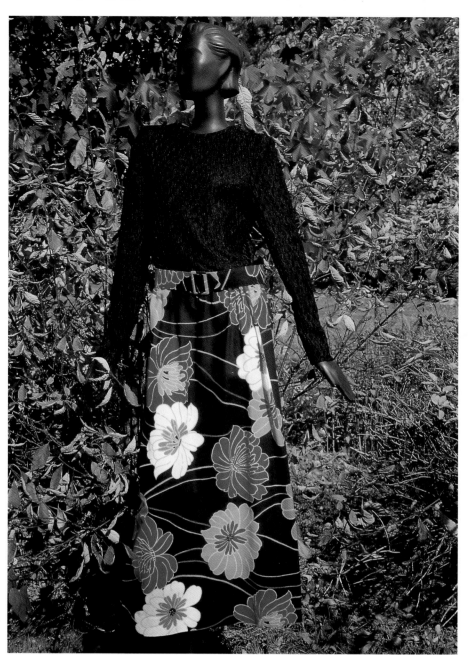

Dress - c. 1960s
I. Magnin & Co.
Black bodice and floral skirt,
100% polyester knit, round
neckline, long sleeve, belted.
$60-$80
Courtesy Studio Moderne

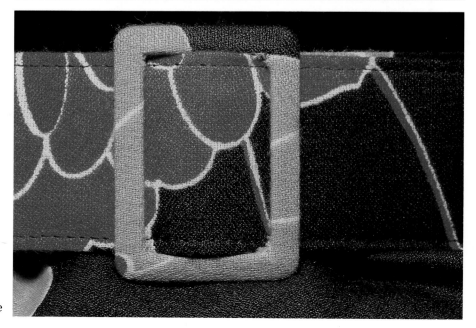

Detail of belt buckle

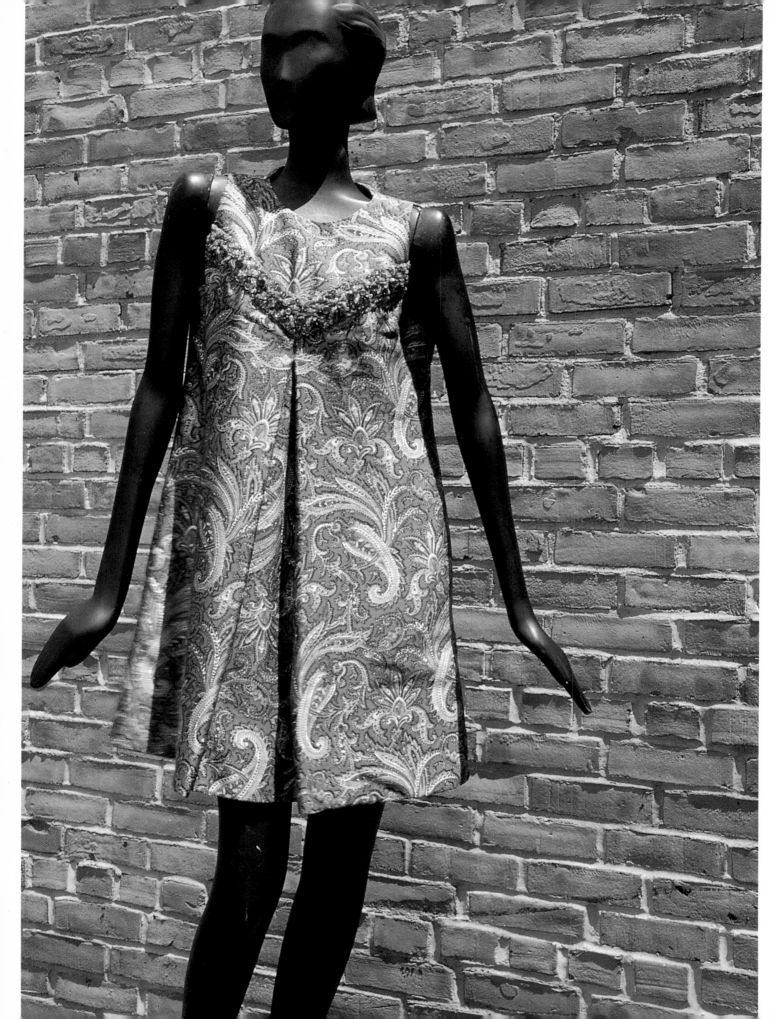

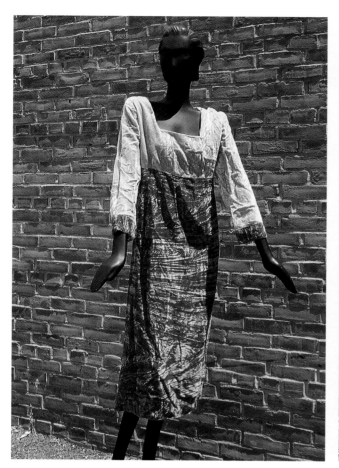

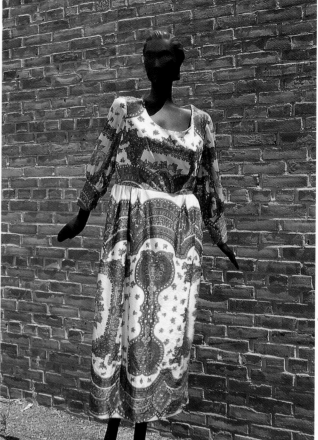

Above:
Dress - c. 1960s
Wine velvet, tie dye, scoop
neckline, trumpet sleeve, empire
waistline.
$50-$75
Courtesy Shelley Stahlman

Above right:
Dress - c. 1960s
Cream 100% polyester bold print,
scoop neckline, long sleeve,
gathered long skirt.
$40-$60
Courtesy Shelley Stahlman

Right:
Dress - c. 1960s
Purple 100% polyester, mini length,
round neckline, long sleeve, eyelet
lacing, empire waistline.
$40-$60
Courtesy Shelley Stahlman

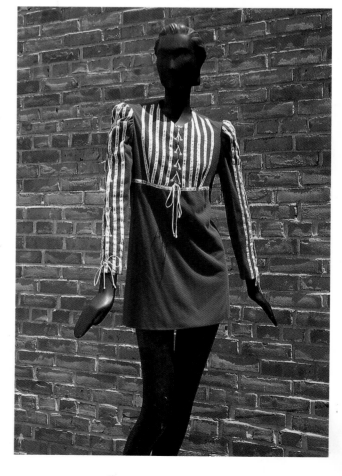

Opposite:
Dress - 1970
Malcolm Starr silk paisley print,
round neckline, sleeveless,
jewel-encrusted trim.
$100-150

Chapter 2

Ensembles

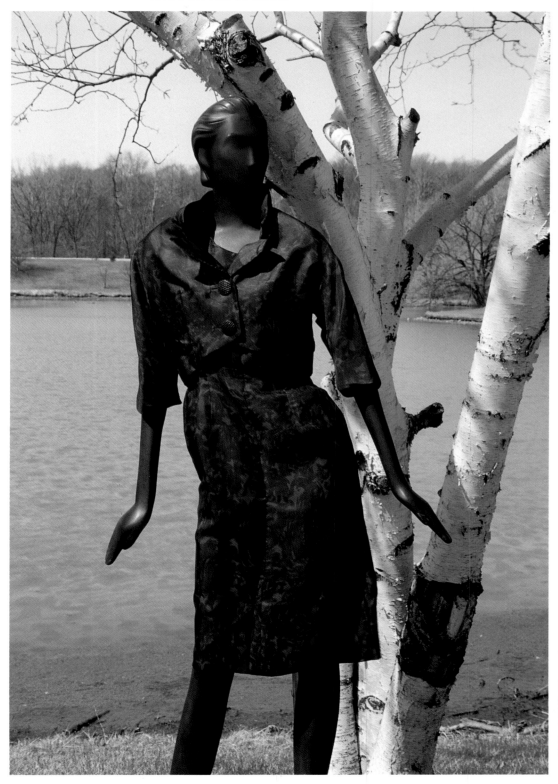

Dress and jacket -
c. 1950s
Blue and black
100% silk, notched
collar, 3/4 sleeve.
$75-$100

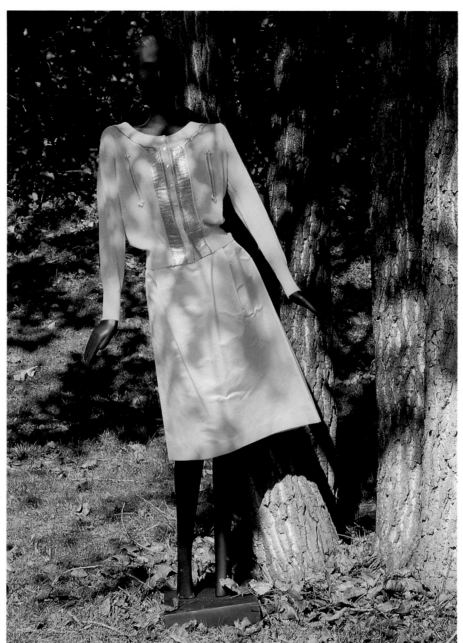

Sweater and skirt -
c. 1950s
Yellow 100% wool
sweater; yellow
satin skirt with gold
ribbon trim.
$70-$90

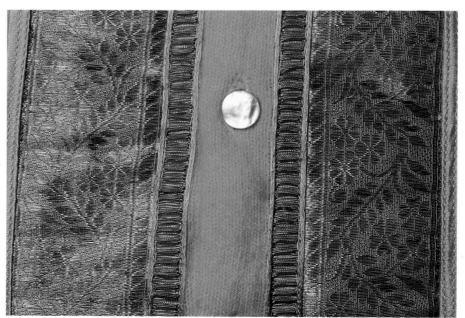

Detail

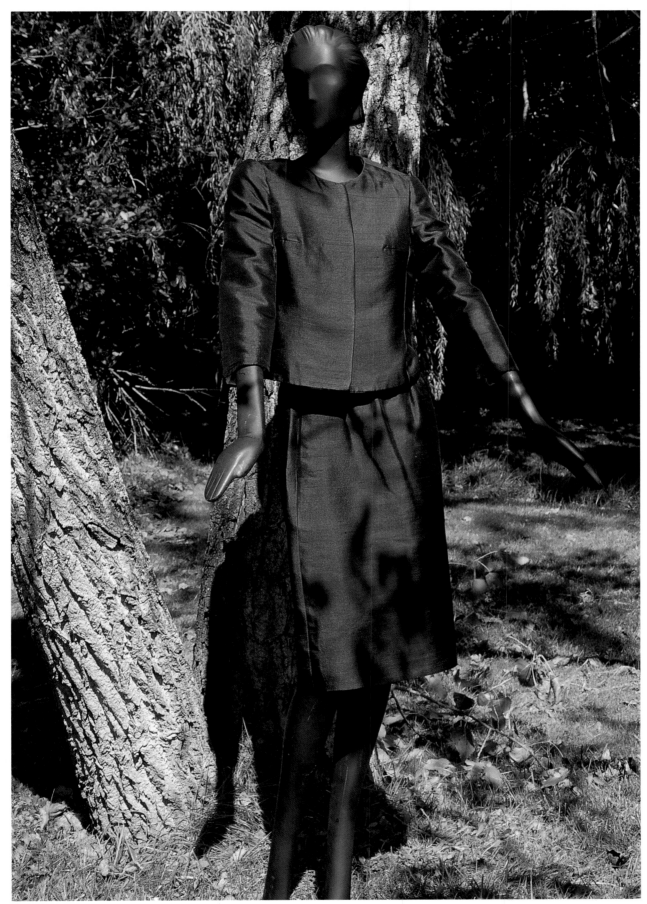

Suit - c. 1950s
Hathaway, Shaker Square
Black 100% silk, box jacket, straight skirt.
$75-$100

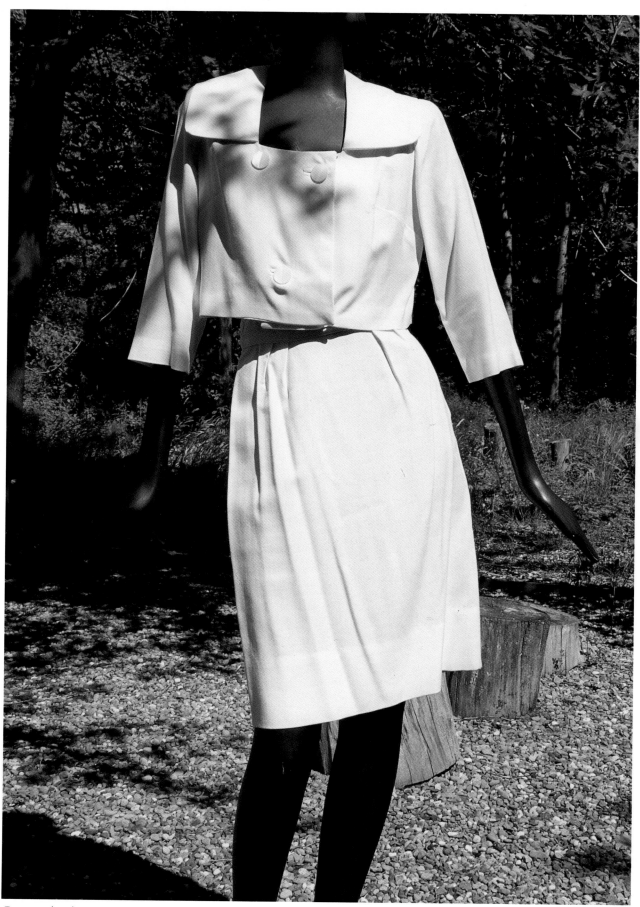

Dress and jacket - c. 1950s
Cream 100% polyester, square
neckline, 3/4 sleeve, gathered skirt.
$50-$75

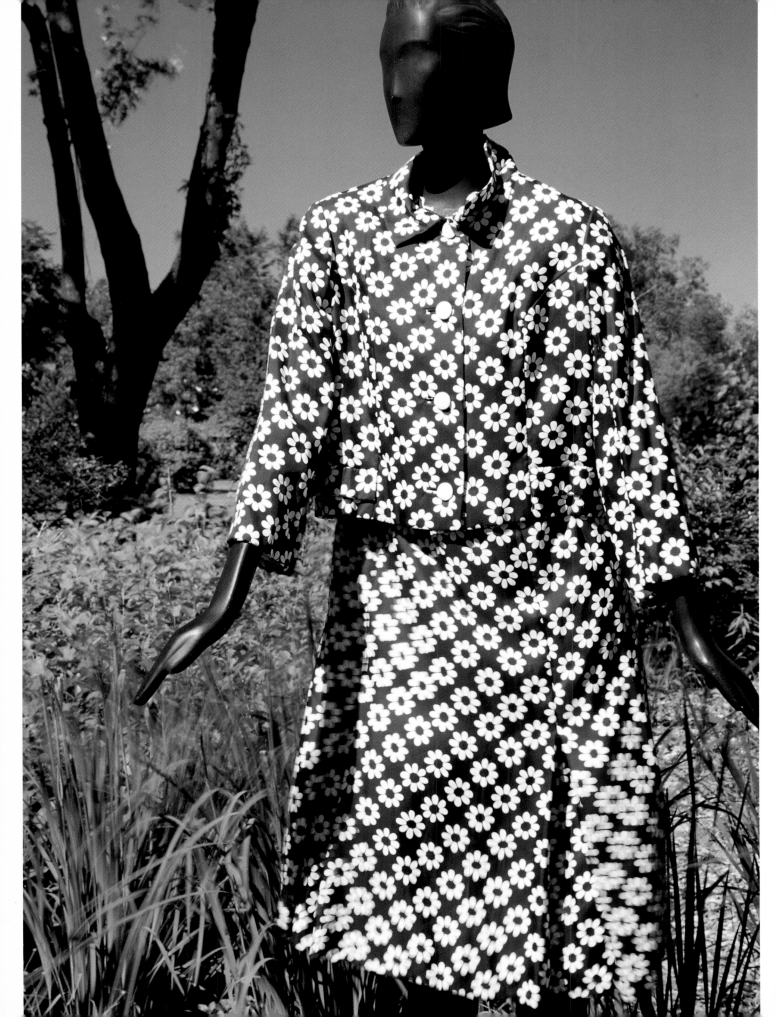

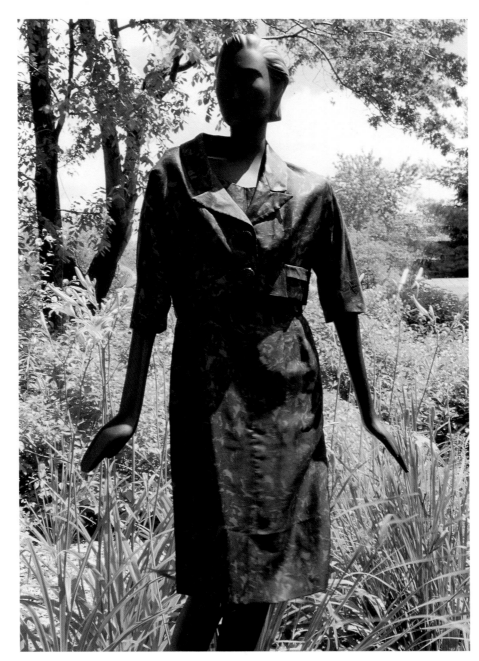

Dress and jacket -
c. 1950s
Purple 100% silk,
notched collar, 3/4
sleeve, large
button and sheath
dress.
$75-$100

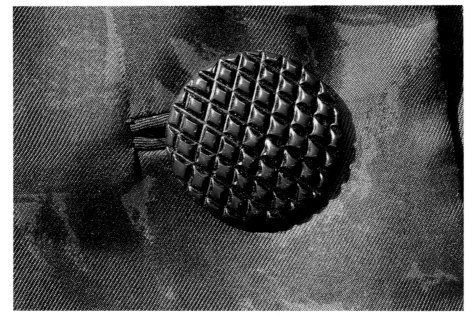

Opposite:
Dress and jacket - c.
1959
Zona Fink Incorpo-
rated, Shaker Heights
Navy 100% silk daisy
print, A-line silhou-
ette, box pleat hem.
$50-$75

Detail of button

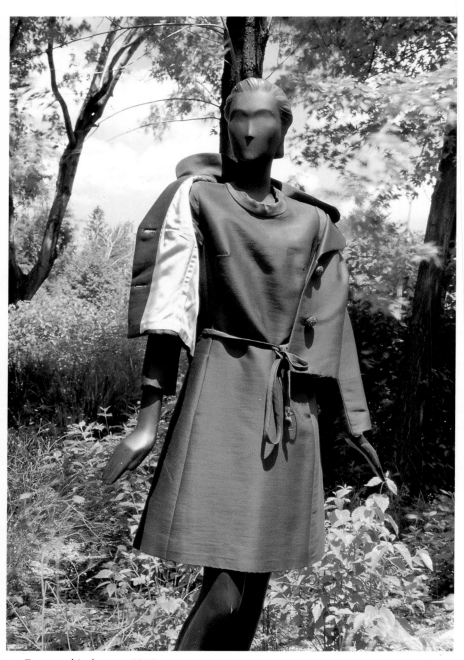

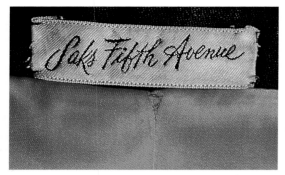

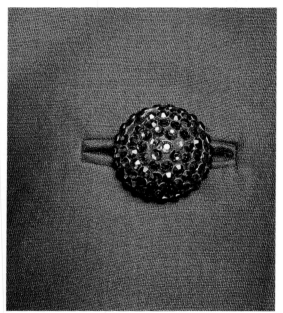

Top:
Label

Above:
Detail of button

Dress and jacket - c. 1950s
Saks Fifth Avenue
Green 100% silk, rounded collar,
princess jacket, rhinestone buttons
and princess panel sheath dress.
$100-$125

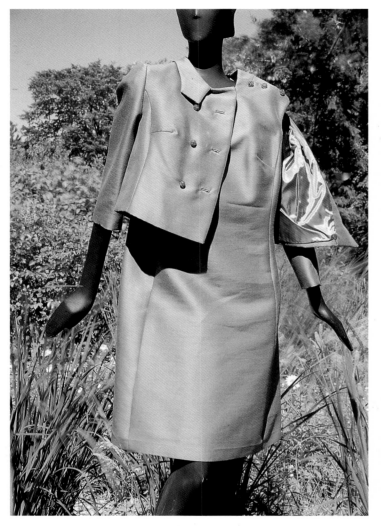

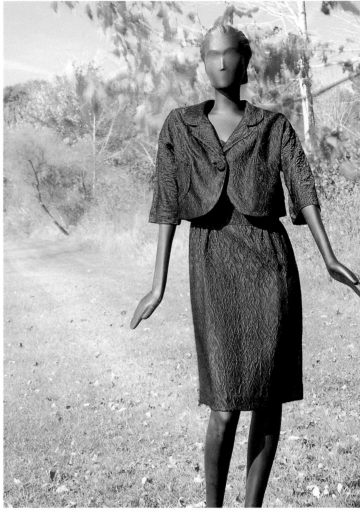

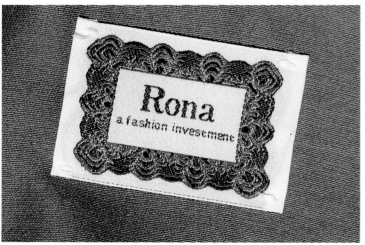

Above left:
Dress and jacket - c. 1950s
Rona
Brown 100% silk, double
breasted jacket, 3/4 sleeve,
rhinestone button and sheath
dress.
$100-$125

Left:
Label

Above right:
Dress and jacket - c. 1950s
Black 100% rayon, notched
collar, large button.

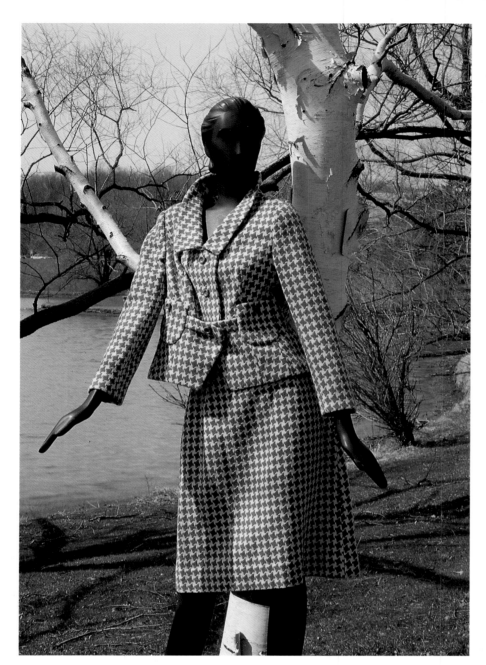

Suit - c. 1950s
Elite Juniors, Styled
by Luba
Brown 100% wool
hound's-tooth
pattern, patch
pockets.
$75-$100

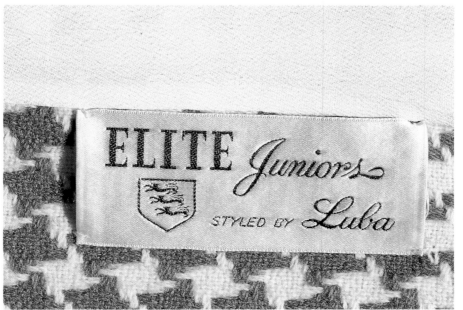

Label

Opposite:
Suit - c. 1960s
Adolphe Zelinka Inc.,
New York
Grey twill 100% wool,
lamb trim collar and cuff.
$150-$175

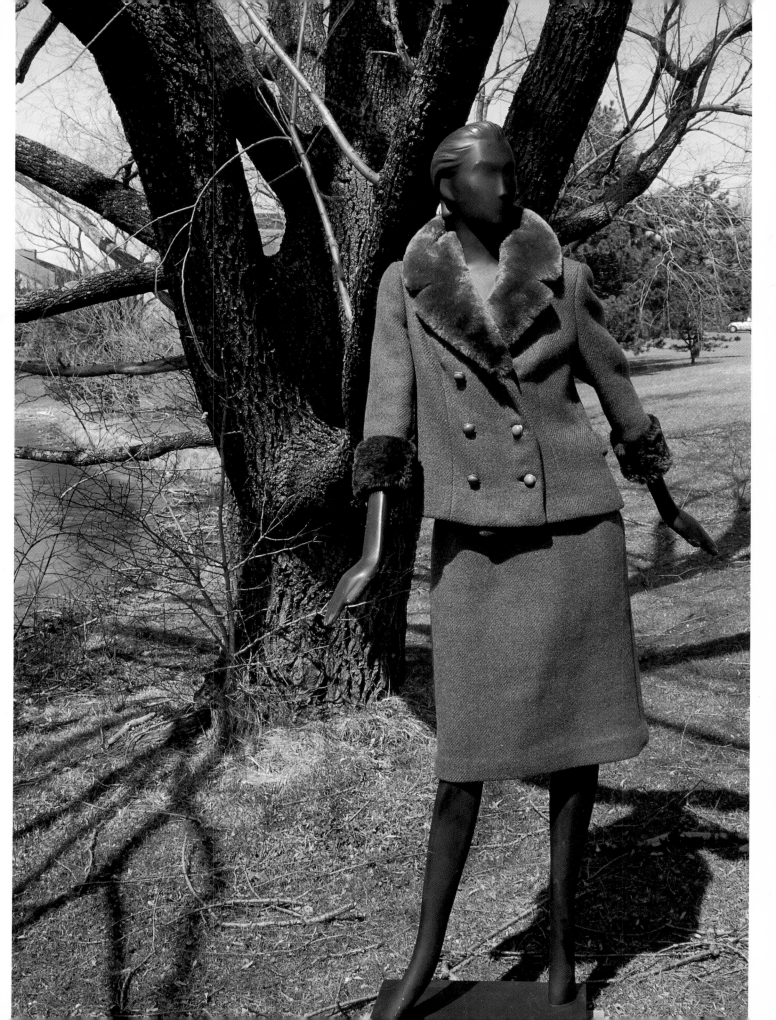

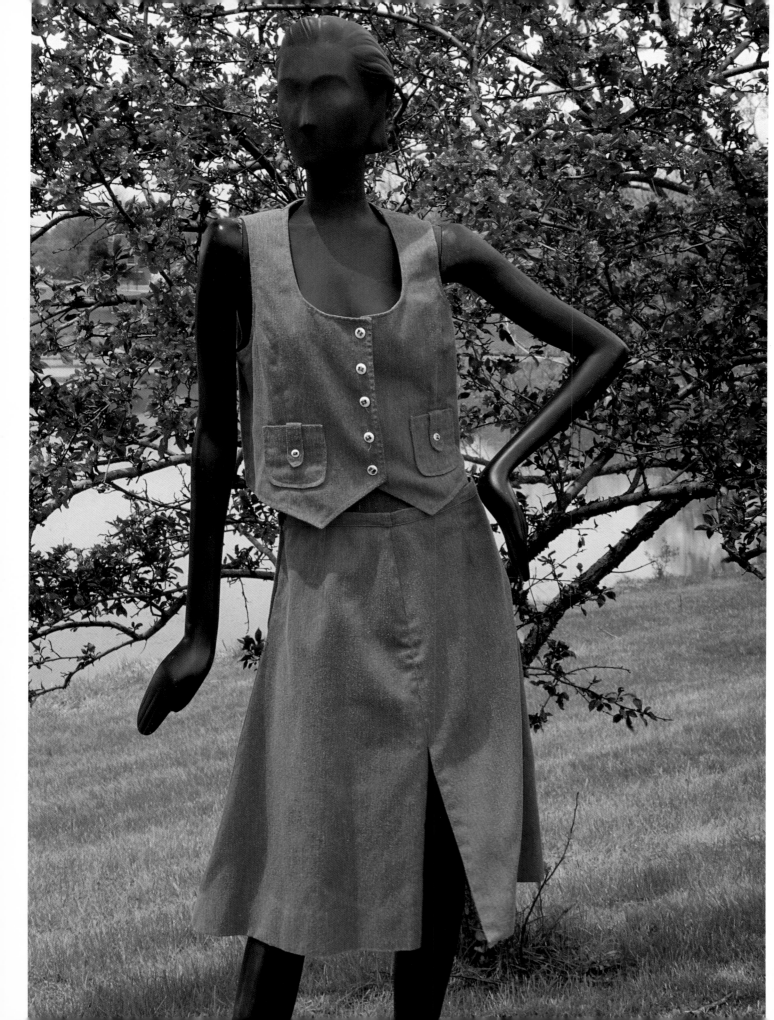

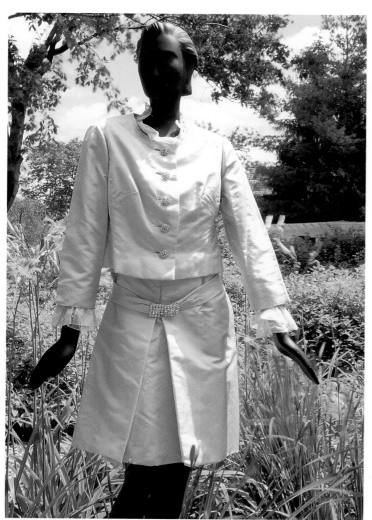

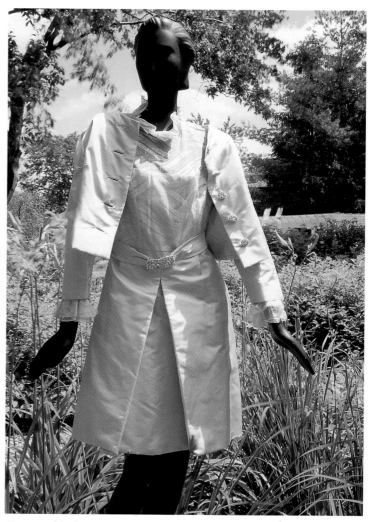

Dress and jacket - c. 1960s
Mignon — Paris, New York
Cream 100% silk, round neckline
jacket, rhinestone button, ruffle bodice,
front pleat skirt with rhinestone belt.
$75-$100

Dress and jacket

Opposite:
Skirt and vest - c. 1970
Blue denim 100% cotton,
scoop neckline fitted vest,
sleeveless, matching skirt;
designed by Shirley Friedland.
$40-$60
Courtesy Shirley Friedland

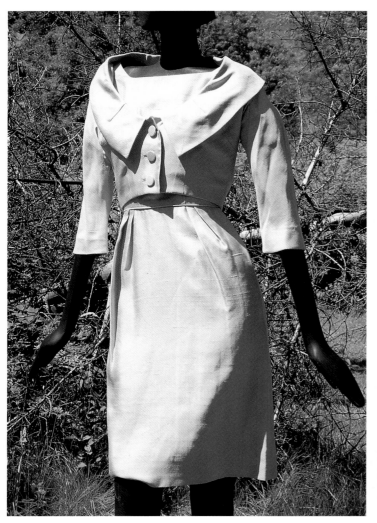

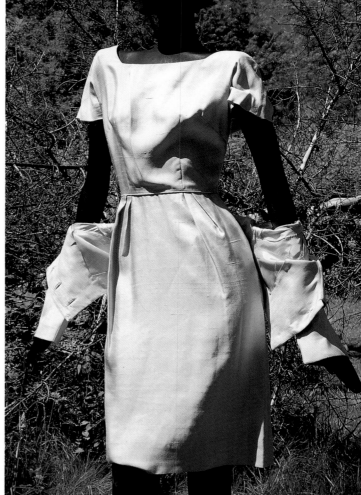

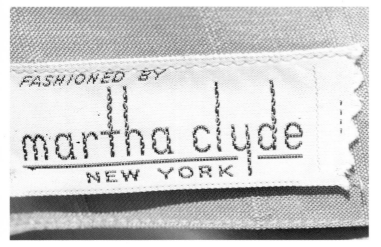

Above left:
Dress and jacket - c. 1961
Fashioned by Martha Clyde, New York
Gold 100% silk, cowl collar, 3/4 sleeve
on jacket and sheath dress.
$75-$100
Courtesy May Brown Korosec

Above right:
Dress and jacket

Left:
Label

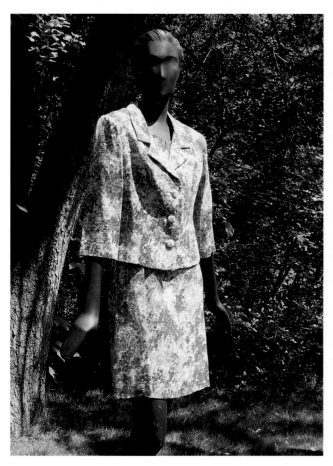

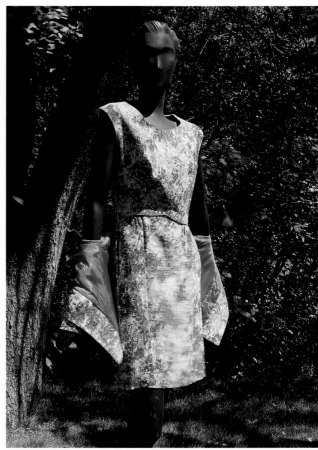

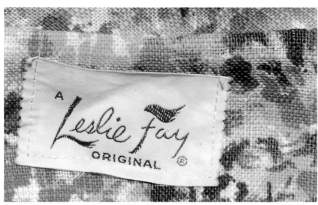

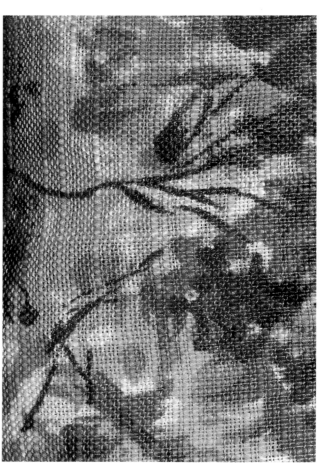

Top left:
Dress and jacket - c. 1966
Leslie Fay Original
Multi 100% linen print, notched
collar, 3/4 sleeve, button jacket
and sheath dress.
$70-$90
Courtesy May Brown Korosec

Top right:
Dress and jacket

Above:
Label

Right:
Detail of fabric

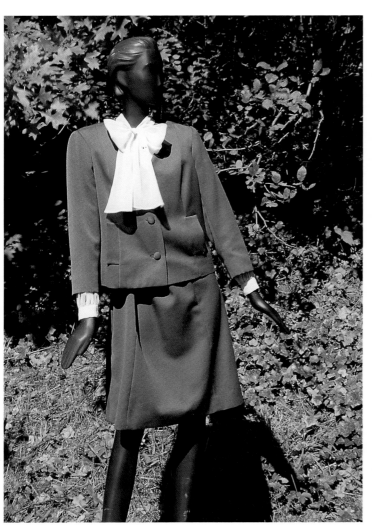

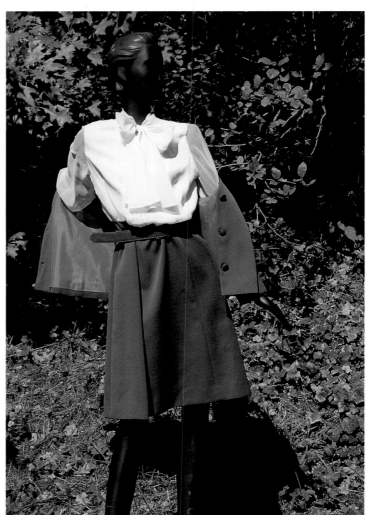

Dress and jacket - c. 1960s
Rona, New York
Grey silk, cream bow
bodice, belted.
$70-90

Dress and jacket

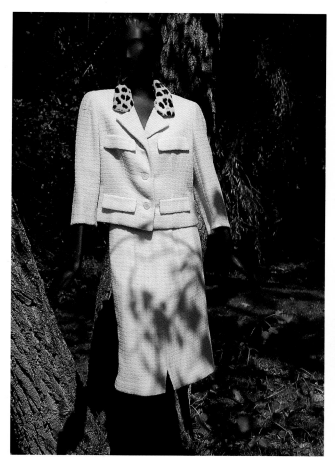

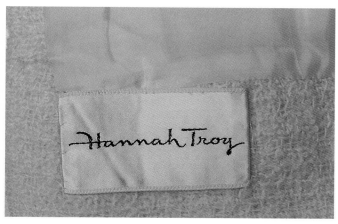

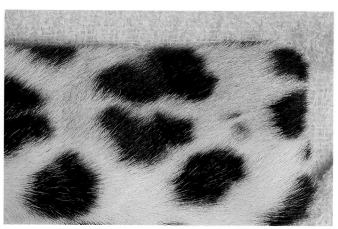

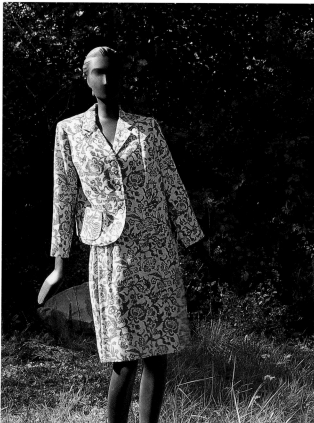

Above left:
Suit - c. 1960s
Hannah Troy
Cream 100% wool, leopard
trim collar.
$100-$150

Top right:
Label

Above:
Detail of leopard collar

Left:
Suit - c. 1966
Peerless of Boston
Cream print, 100% linen,
notched collar, straight skirt.
$50-$75

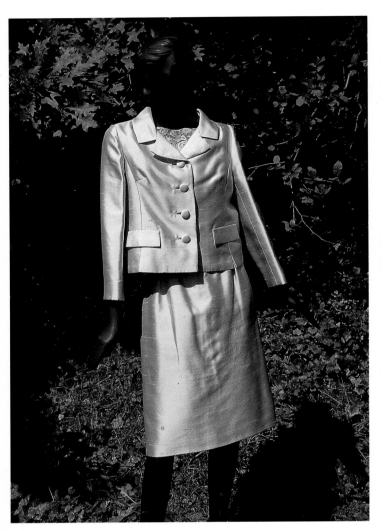

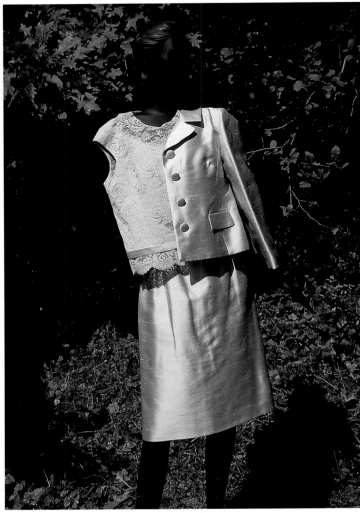

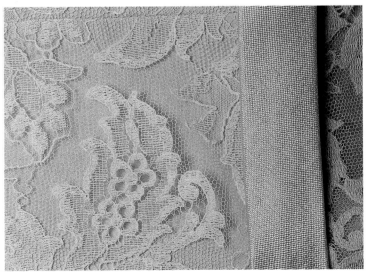

Above left:
Suit - c. 1960s
Grey 100% silk, notched collar,
flap pocket, lace bodice.
$75-$100

Above right:
Suit

Left:
Detail of lace

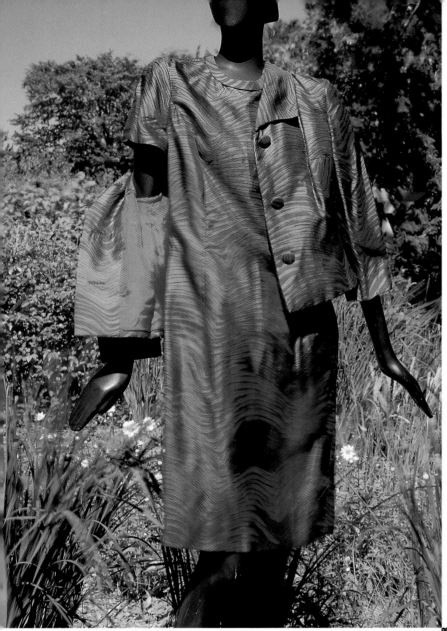

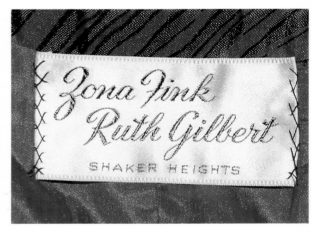

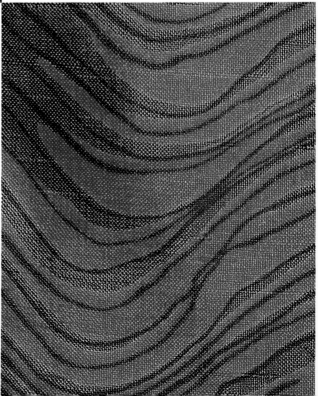

Above:
Dress and Jacket - c. 1960s
Zona Fink
Red and brown 100% silk
print, collar, 3/4 sleeve,
button, jacket, sheath dress.
$75-$100

Above right:
Label

Right:
Detail of fabric

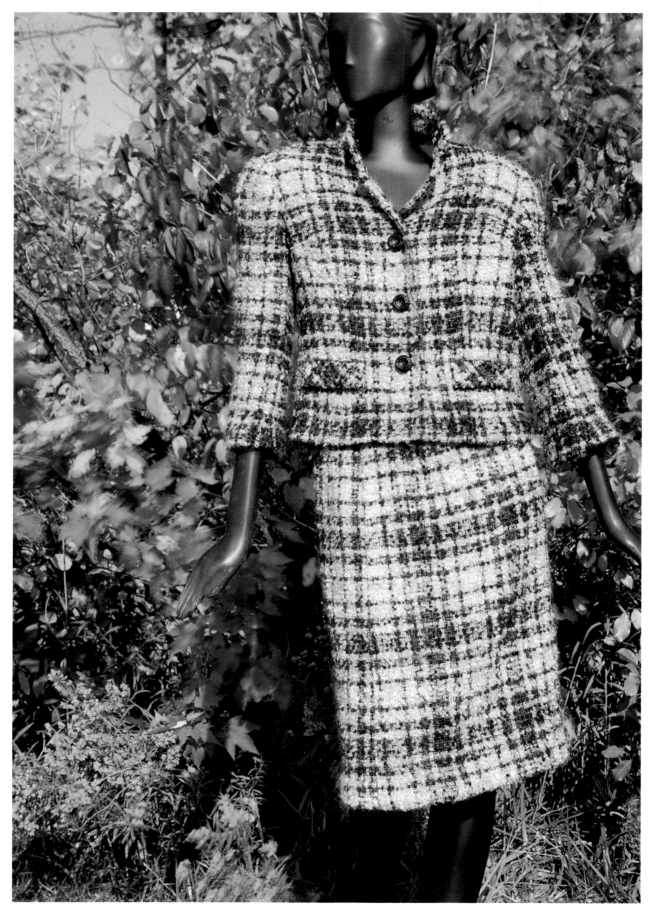

Suit - c. 1960s
Davidow — London, Paris, New York
Brown plaid 100% mohair wool,
notched collar, flap pocket.
$60-$80

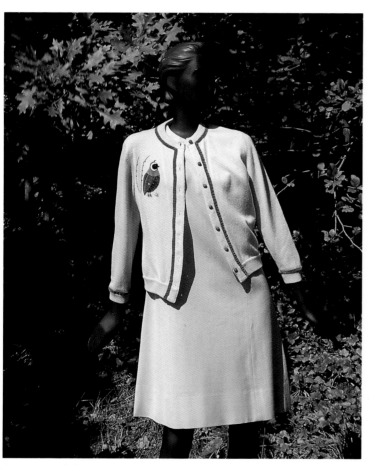

Sweater and dress - c. 1950s
Lee Collins sweater; Dalton dress
Beige 100% wool, velvet quail appliqué.
$50-$75

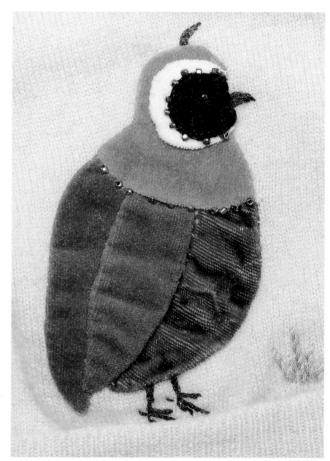

Detail of quail appliqué

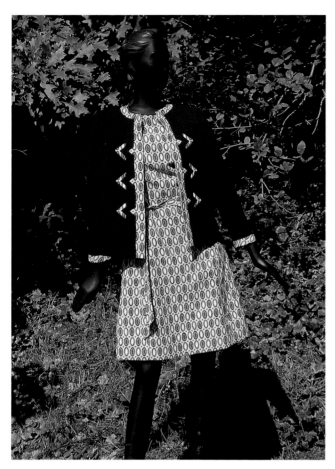

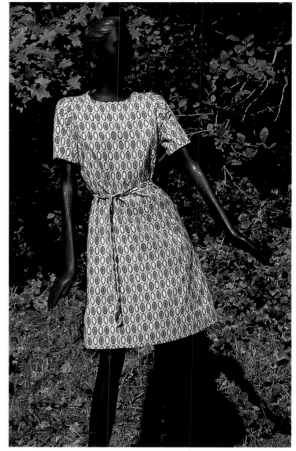

Above:
Sweater and dress -
c. 1950s
Navy sweater, 100%
wool; print dress,
100% silk.
$70-$90

Above right:
Dress

Right:
Detail

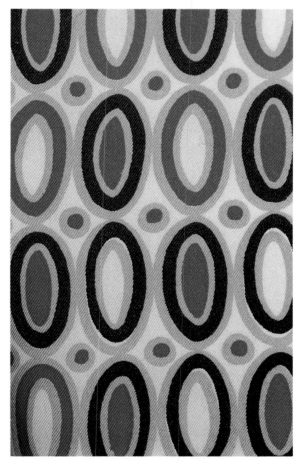

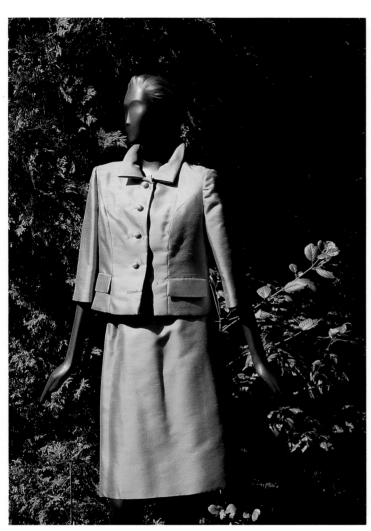

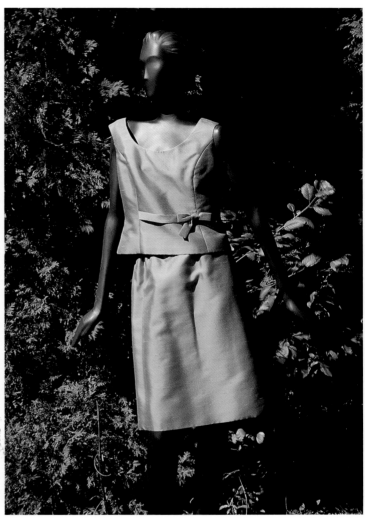

Suit - c. 1959
Milgrim
Apple green 100% silk, flap
pocket, belted shell, straight skirt.
$75-$100

Shell and skirt

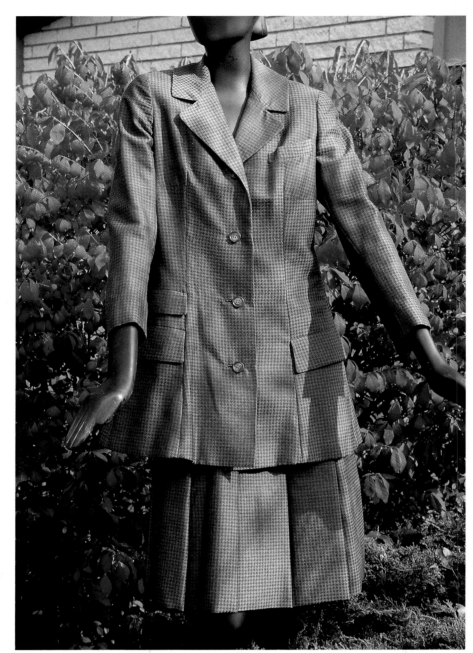

Suit - c. 1952
Zelinka Matliek — New
York, London, Paris
Grey and blue silk and
mohair, notched collar,
long torso jacket, box
pleat skirt.
$150-$175
*Courtesy Shirley
Friedland*

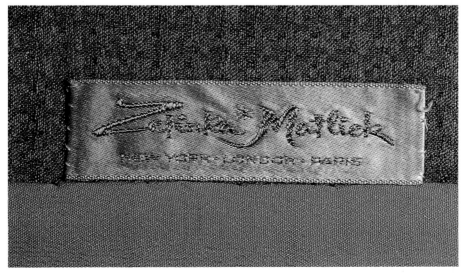

Label

Sweater and dress - c. 1950s
Aqua sweater, 100% wool; aqua dress,
100% silk, bow appliqué, spaghetti belt.
$50-$75

Sweater and dress

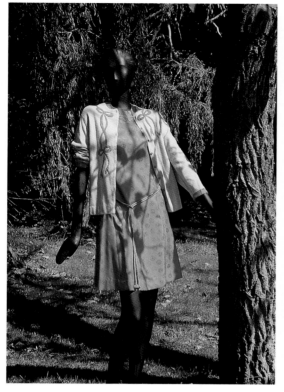

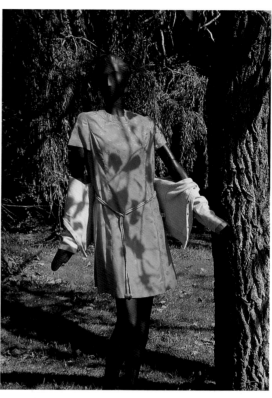

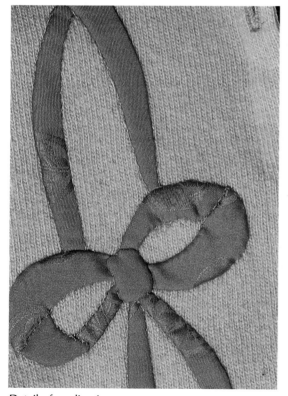

Detail of appliqué

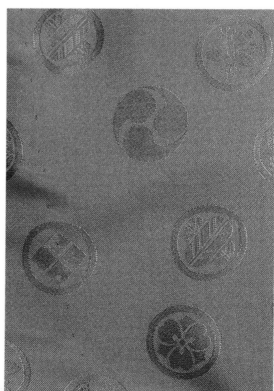

Detail of fabric

Suit - c. 1950s
Black pattern 100% silk,
velvet collar, crochet button.
$70-$90

Suit - c. 1950s
Bonwit Teller Country Place
Navy 100% wool, round
collar, straight skirt.
$70-$90

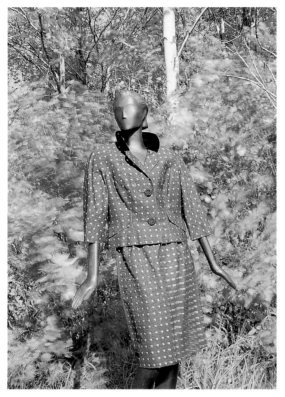

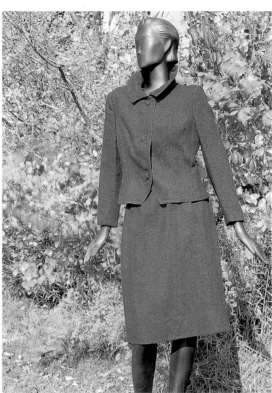

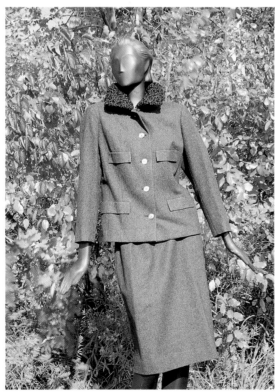

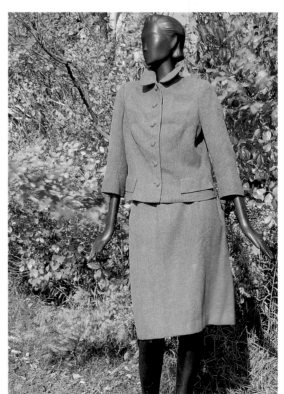

Suit - c. 1950s
Jaeger, London
Grey 100% wool, lamb collar,
flap pocket, straight skirt.
$100-$150

Suit - c. 1950s
Grey 100% wool, flap
pocket, straight skirt.
$70-$90

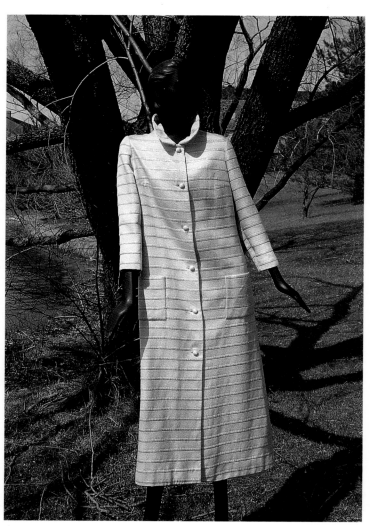

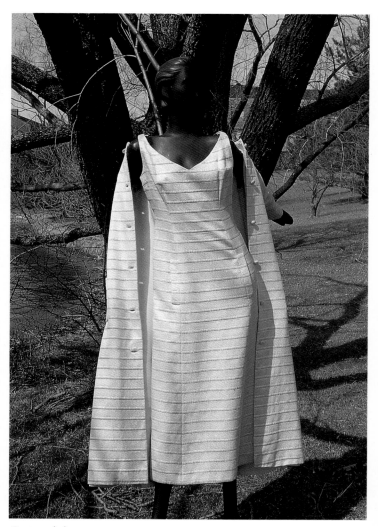

Coat and dress - c. 1960s
Silver lamé 100% silk,
patch pocket.
$100-$150

Coat and dress

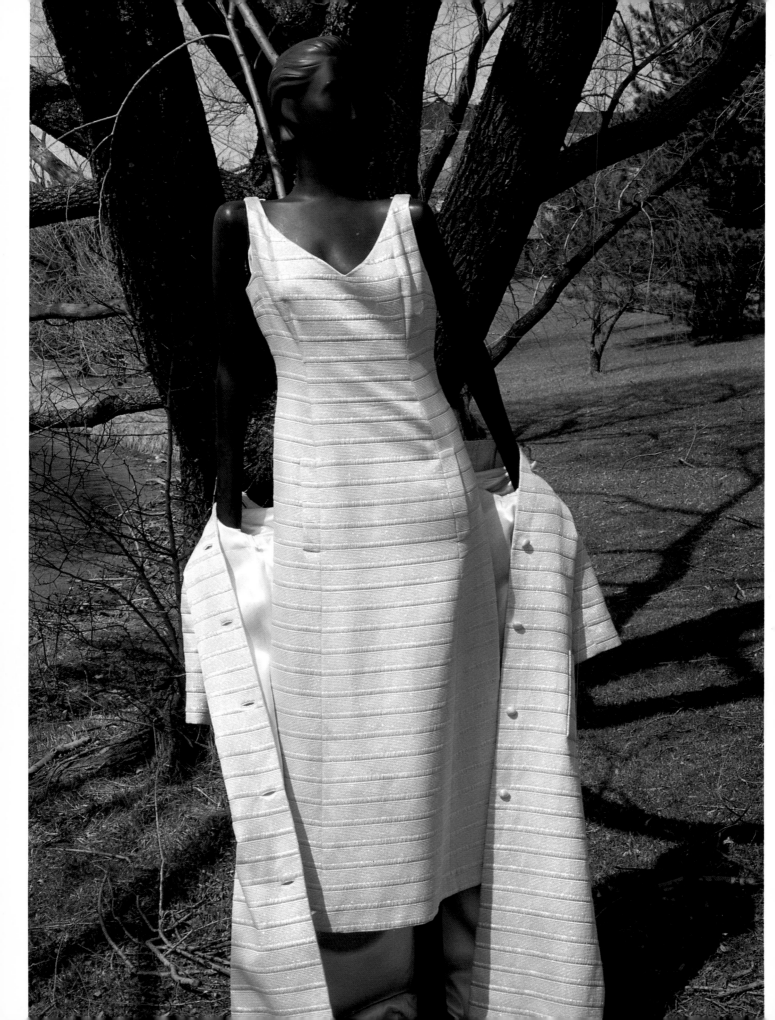

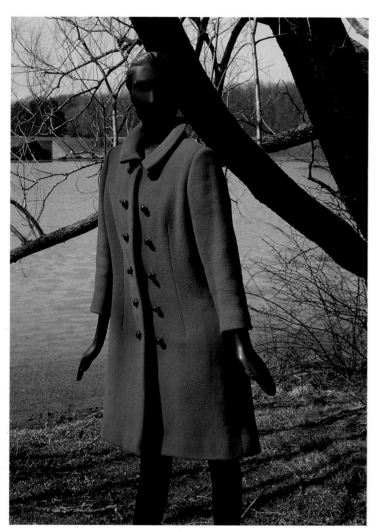 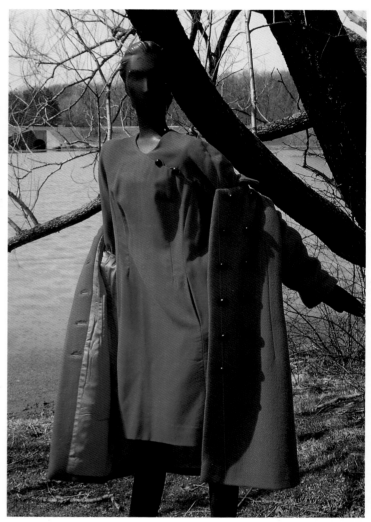

Coat and dress - c. 1960s
Aqua 100% wool, double
breasted, sheath silhouette.
$75-$100

Coat and dress

Opposite:
Dress only, from page 81

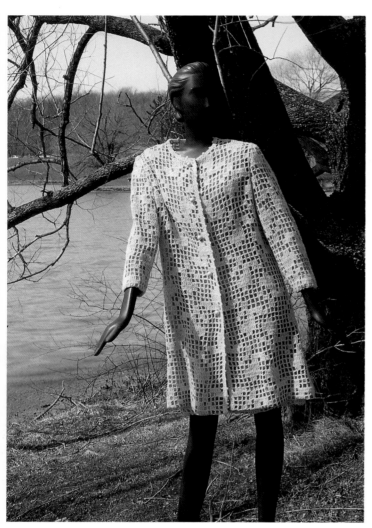

Coat and dress - c. 1960s
Yellow 100% silk, crochet
coat and dress.
$75-$125

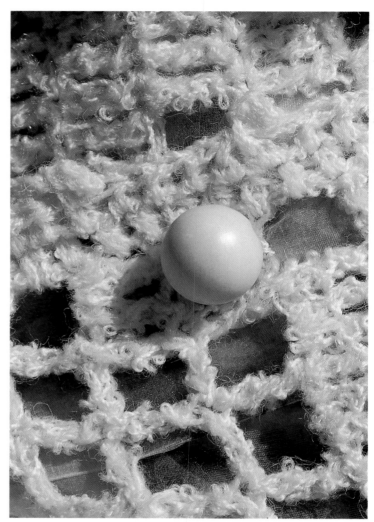

Detail of fabric

Opposite:
Coat and dress

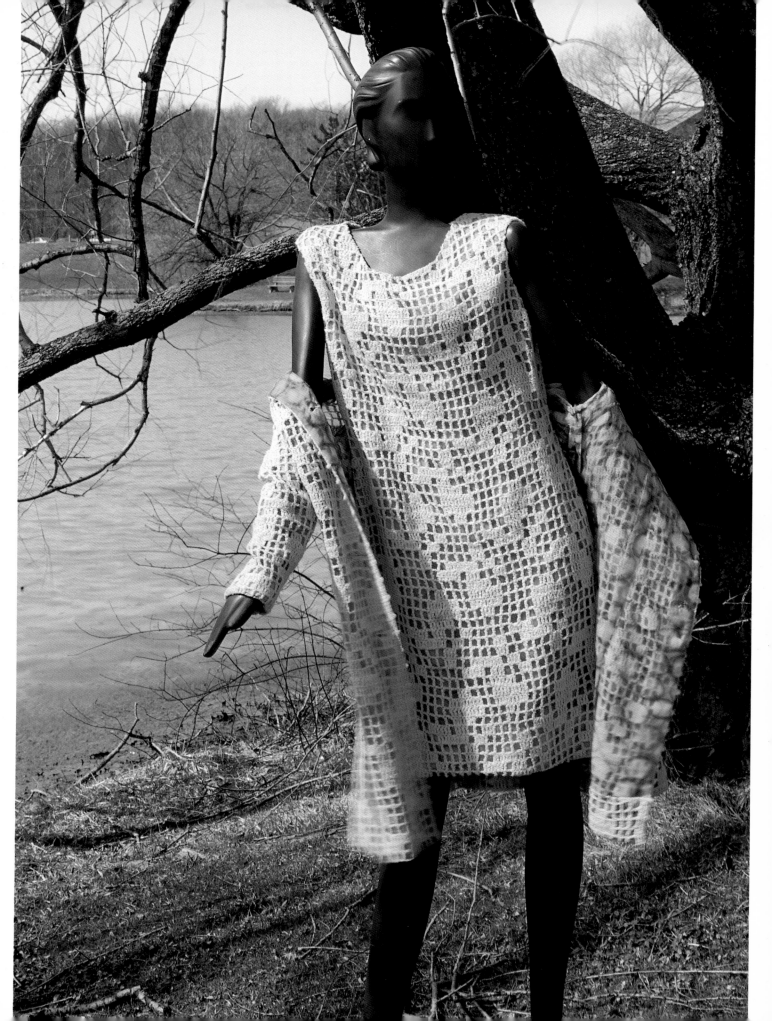

Coat and dress - c. 1960s
Beige 100% polyester knit,
double breasted, flap pocket.
$50-$75

Coat and dress

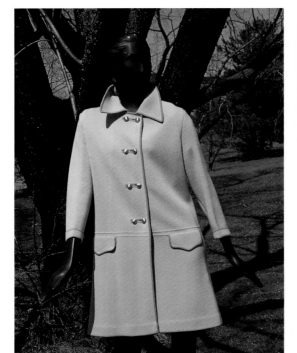

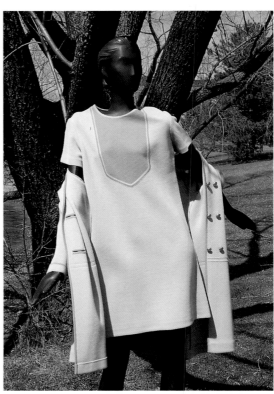

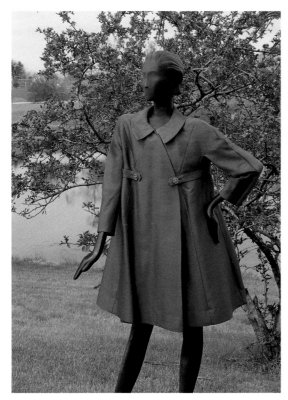

Coat and dress - c. 1960s
Logan Knitting Mills, Logan, Utah
Green 100% silk, empire coat and dress.
$75-$100

Coat and dress

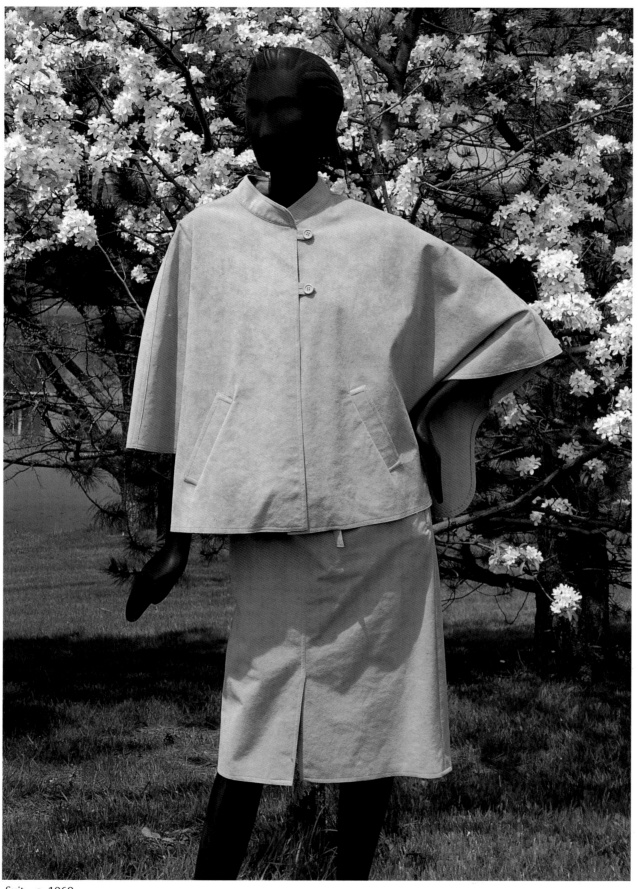

Suit - c. 1969
Joan Leslie by Kasper
Peach 100% Skinner ultra suede,
slim skirt with dramatic cape.
$100-$150
Courtesy Shirley Friedland

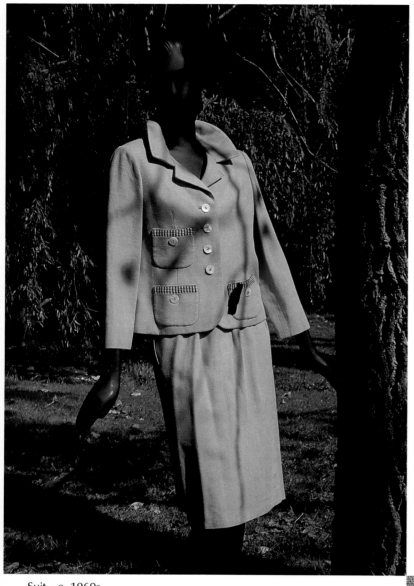

Suit - c. 1960s
Orange 100% linen, notched
collar, patch pocket.
$70-$90

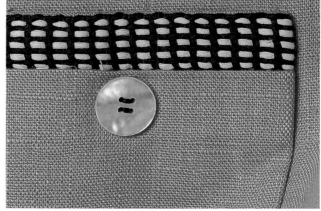

Detail of pocket

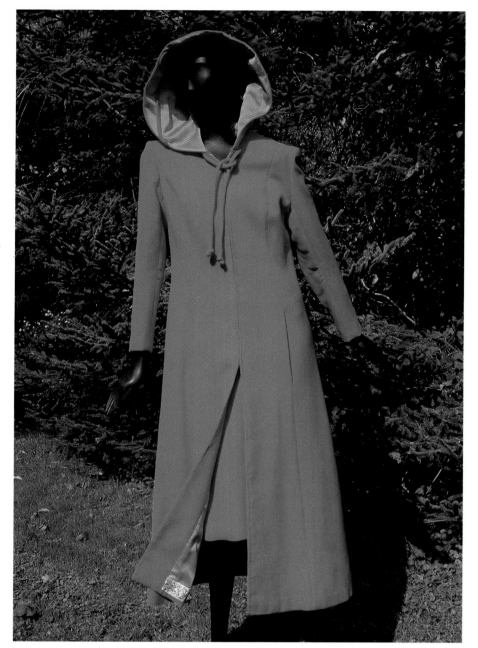

Above:
Coat and skirt - c. 1969
Hot pink 100% wool gabardine,
satin lined hood, evening coat
and matching skirt with front
zipper closure; designed by
Shirley Friedland.
$150-$175
Courtesy Shirley Friedland

Left:
Skirt

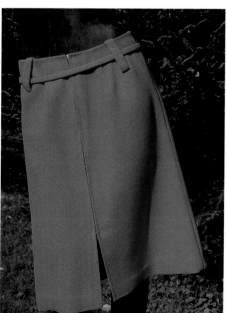

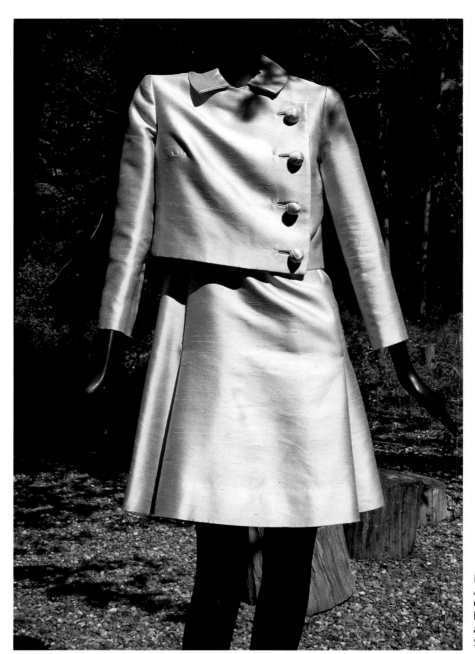

Dress and jacket - c. 1960s
A.F. Boutique, Anne Fogarty
Grey 100% silk, collar, side
button closure, long sleeve
and side seam box pleat.
$100-$150

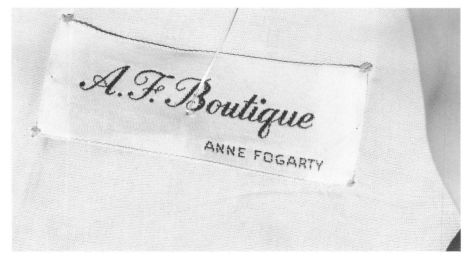

Label

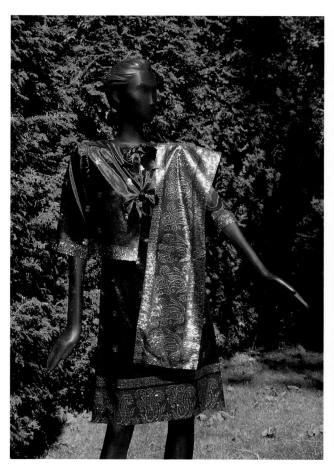

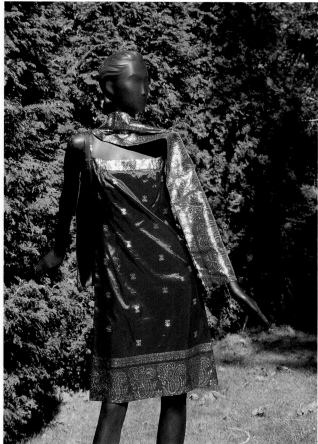

Above:
Jacket/dress/shawl - c. 1960s
Black and silver 100% silk lamé,
3/4 sleeve jacket, sheath dress
and shawl.
$75-$100

Above right:
Dress and shawl

Right:
Detail of fabric

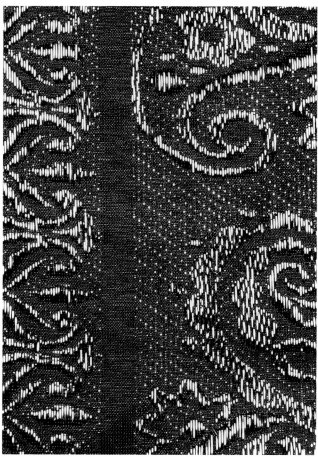

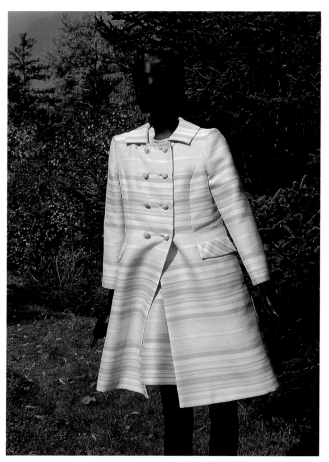

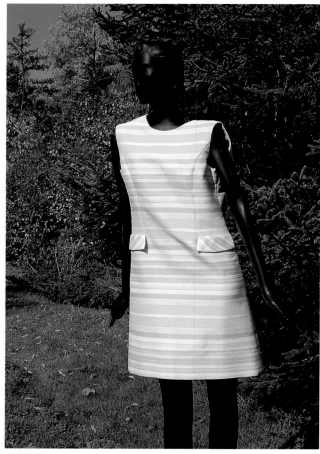

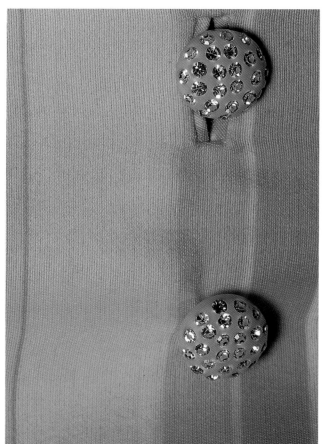

Above left:
Coat and dress - c. 1960s
Evelyn Bader — Paris, Cleveland
Multi-stripe silk and wool, double breasted, long sleeve coat, rhinestone button, sleeveless sheath dress.
$100-$150
Courtesy Studio Moderne

Above:
Dress

Left:
Detail of button

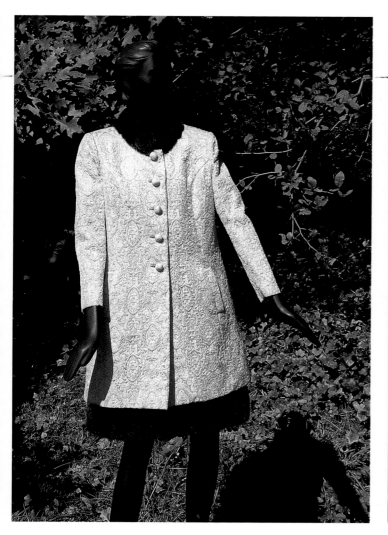

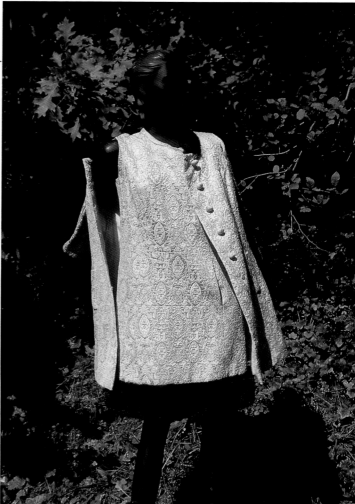

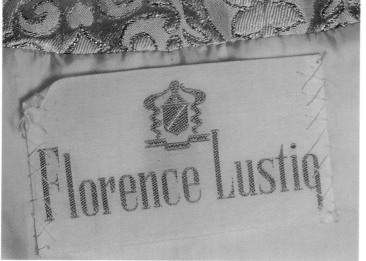

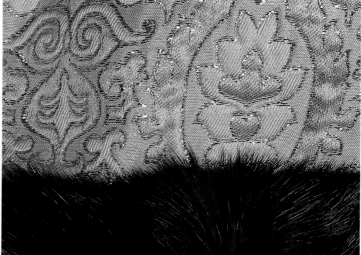

Top:
Coat and dress - c. 1960s
Florence Lustig
Gold 100% silk lamé, mink trim coat
collar and mink trim dress hem.
$175-$225

Bottom:
Label

Top:
Coat and dress

Bottom:
Detail of fabric

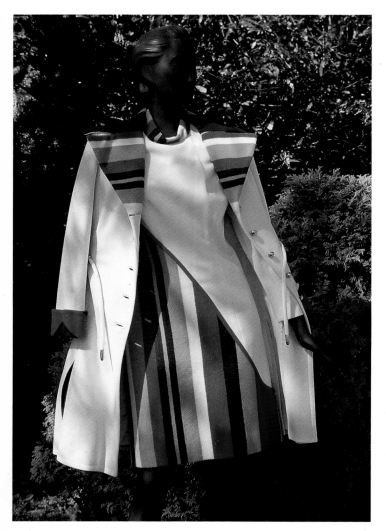

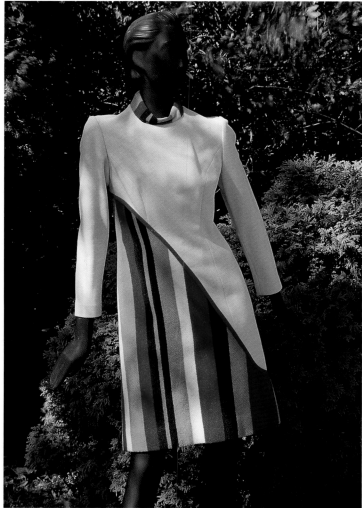

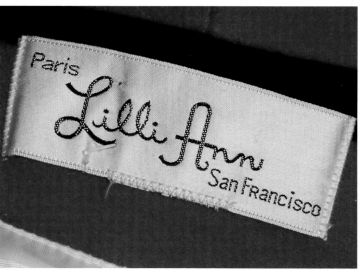

Above left:
Coat and dress - c. 1960s
Lilli Ann — Paris, San Francisco
Cream and multi-color stripe,
polyester knit, notched collar, brass
button.
$100-$150

Above right:
Dress

Left:
Label

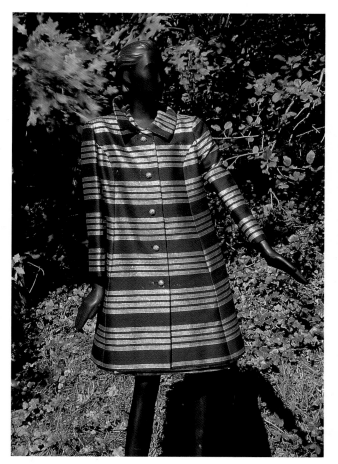

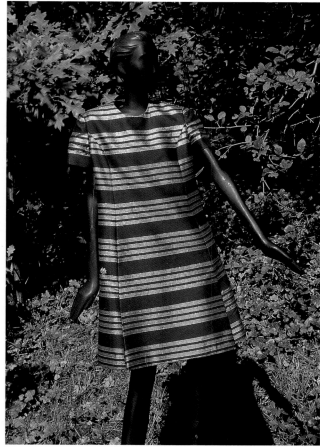

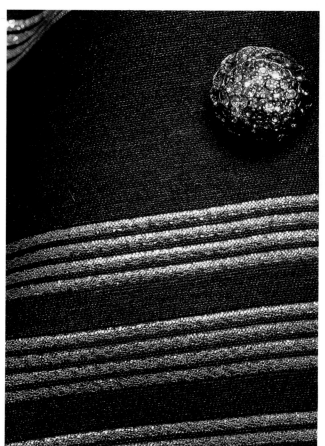

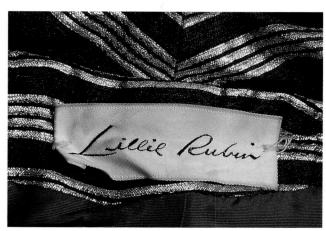

Top left:
Coat and dress - c. 1960s
Lillie Rubin
Navy 100% silk lamé,
rhinestone button.
$100-$150

Top right:
Dress

Left:
Detail of rhinestone button

Above:
Label

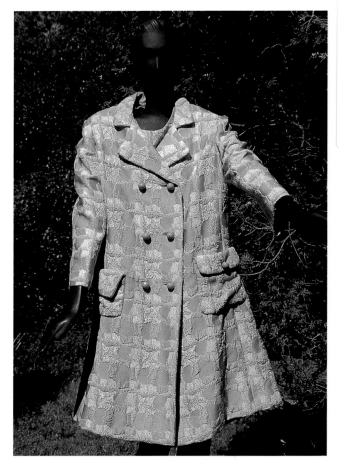

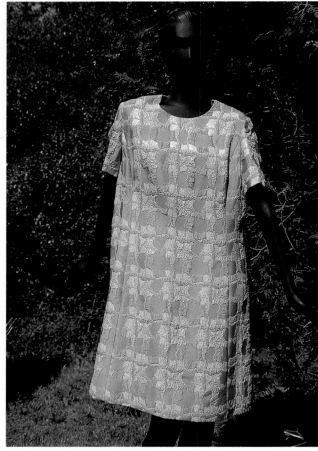

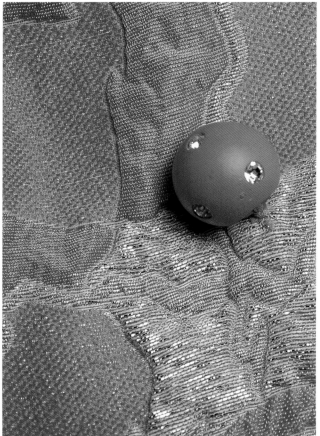

Above left:
Coat and dress - c. 1960s
Pink 100% rayon lamé, notched
lapel, double breasted.
$70-$90

Above right:
Dress

Left:
Detail of rhinestone button

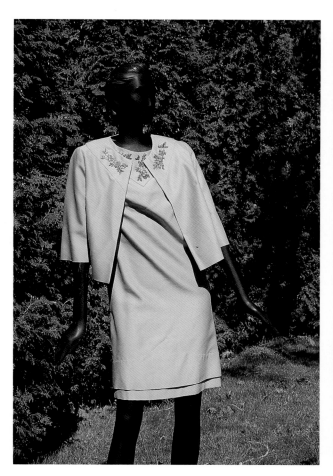

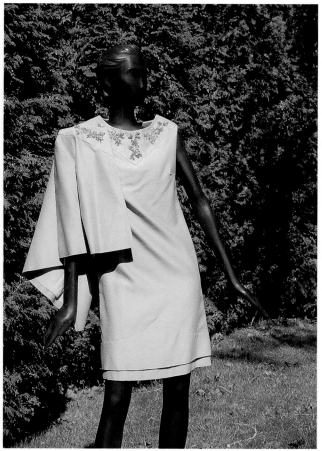

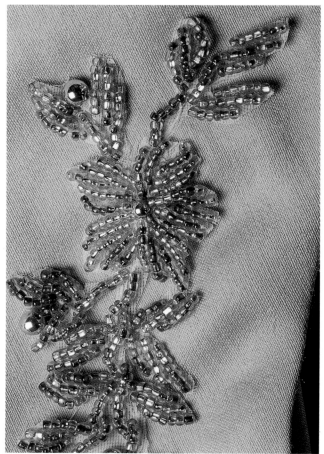

Above:
Jacket and dress - c. 1960s
Green 100% silk, beaded box
jacket, beaded dress yoke.
$100-$125

Above right:
Jacket and dress

Right:
Detail of beading

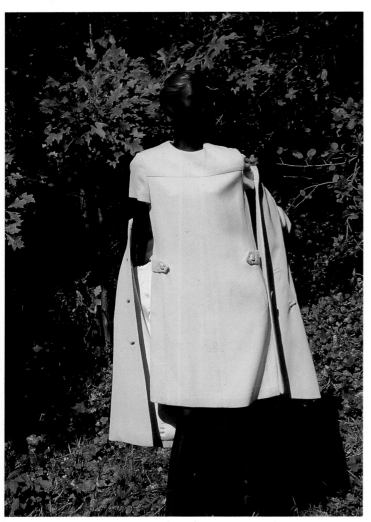

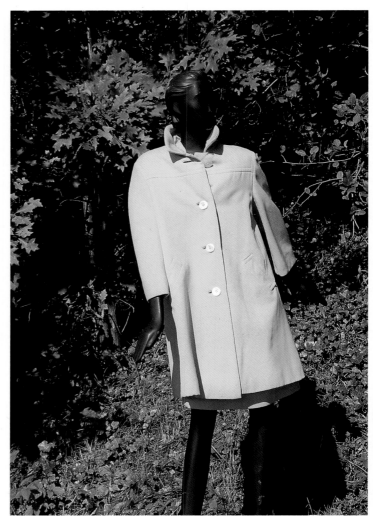

Coat and dress - c. 1960s
Melvine Miller
Yellow gaberdine dress with
hidden pocket and side trim.
$80-120

Coat and dress

Coat and dress - c. 1960s
Arkin Imports, Tailored in British Crown
Colony Hong Kong.
Multi-color silk print, black stone button.
$90-110

Open coat

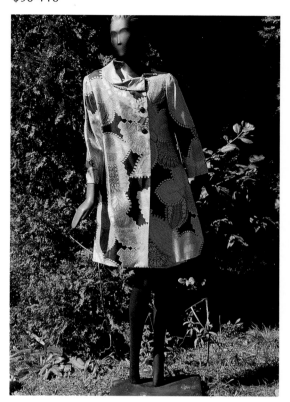
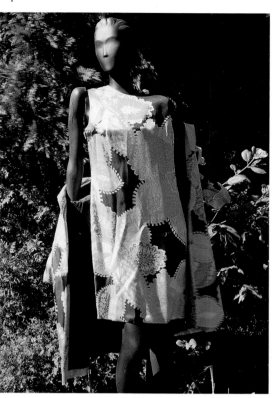

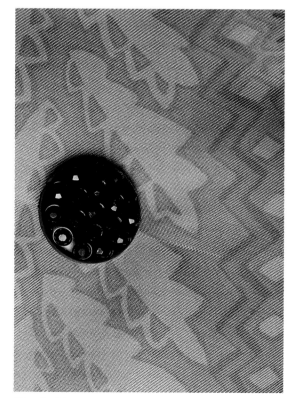
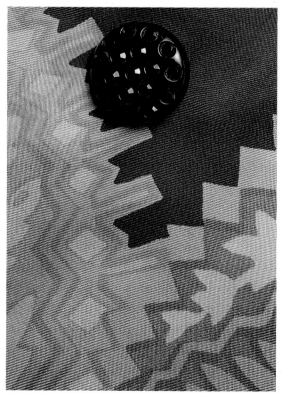

Detail of button

Detail of fabric

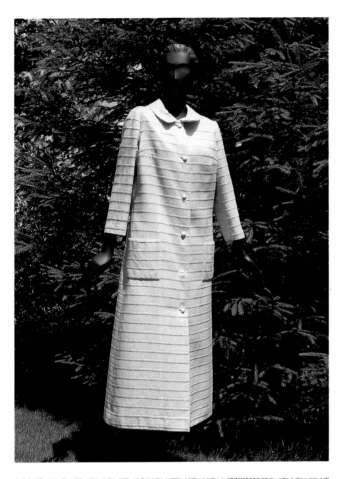

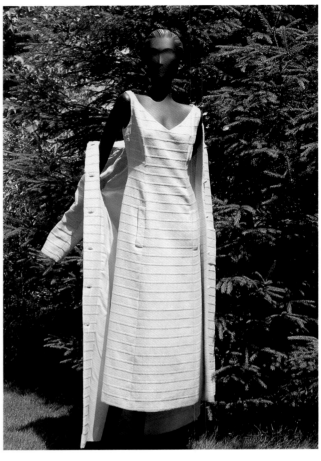

Above left:
Coat and dress - c. 1960s
Silver 100% silk lamé, collar,
long sleeve, patch pocket; dress
V-neckline, sleeveless.
$100-$125

Above right:
Coat and dress

Left:
Detail of fabric

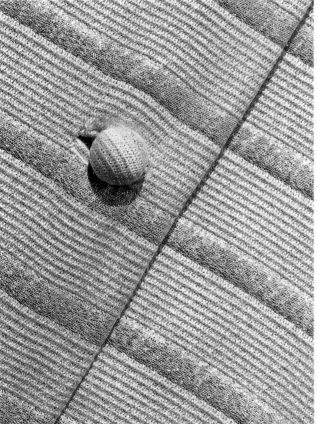

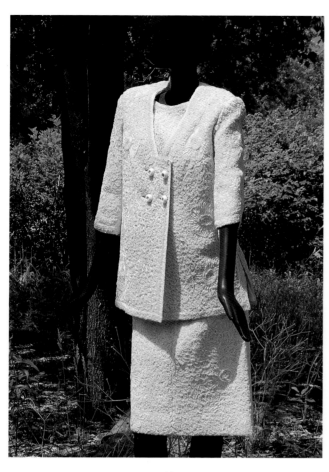

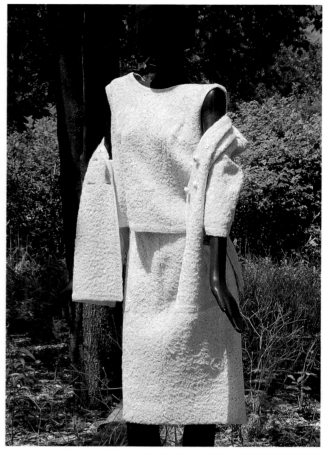

Above:
Jacket, skirt, and shell - c. 1960s
Jack Kobren
Engel-Fetzer Cleveland
Yellow 100% silk ribbon
crochet, 3/4 sleeve, double
breasted, shell, straight skirt.
$100-$150

Above right:
Suit

Right:
Detail of fabric

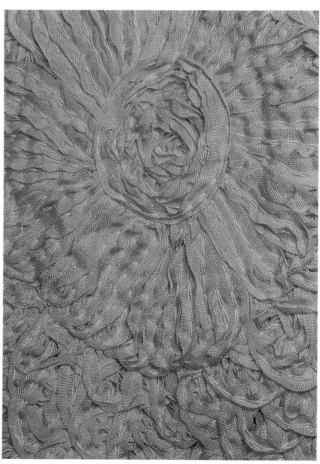

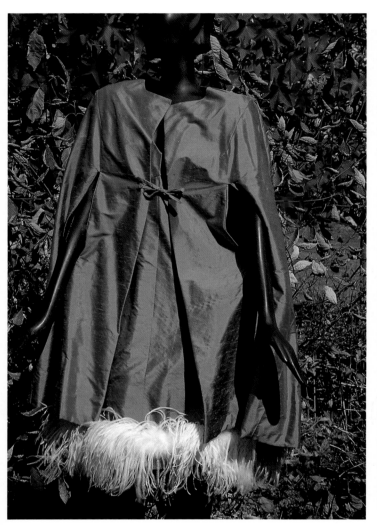

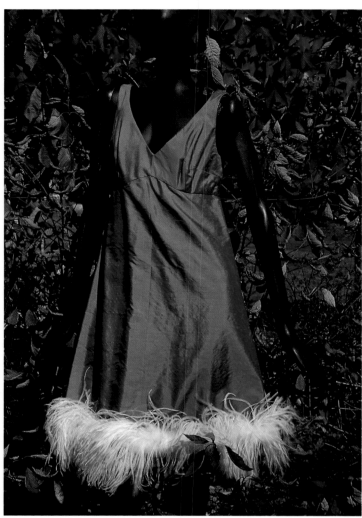

Cape and dress - c. 1965
Turquoise 100% oriental silk, evening
cape with ostrich feather trim on dress
hem; designed by Shirley Friedland.
$200-$225
Courtesy Shirley Friedland

Dress with ostrich feather

Opposite:

Top left: Suit - c. 1960s
Blue and Grey 100% Skinner ultra
suede, hood, belt sash, straight skirt.
$100-$150
Courtesy Shirley Friedland

Top right: Suit - c. 1960s
Floral pattern polyester knit, diagonal
stripe with large flowers, bishop sleeve,
full cut bodice and skirt; designed by
Shirley Friedland.
$40-$60
Courtesy Shirley Friedland

Bottom left: Suit - c. 1960s
Adele Simpson
Mary Louise, Cleveland,
Ohio
Turquoise 100% ultra suede,
round neckline, long sleeve,
straight skirt.
$100-$150
Courtesy Shirley Friedland

Center right: Label

Bottom right: Label

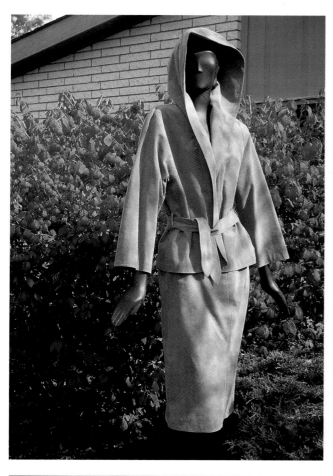

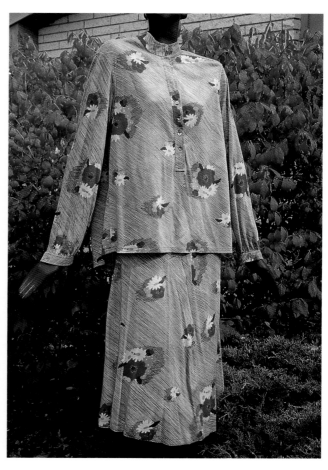

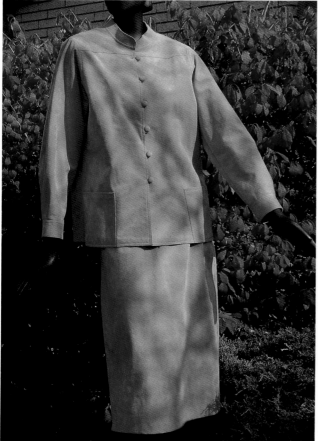

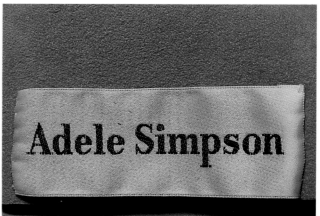

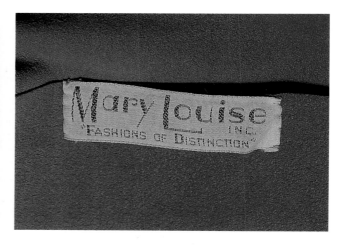

Chapter 3

Sweaters

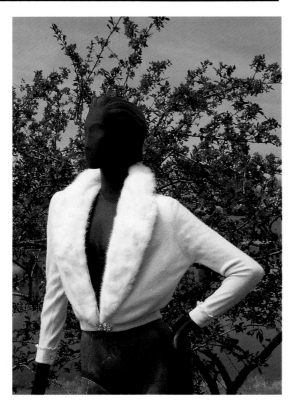

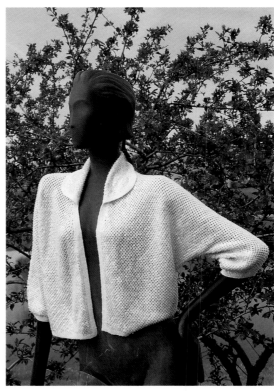

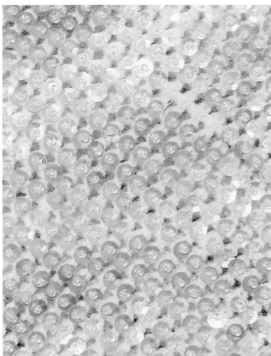

Above left:
Sweater - c. 1955
White 100% cashmere, detachable
mink collar, rhinestone closure.
$100-150
Courtesy Shirley Friedland

Above right:
Sweater - c. 1958
Cream 100% wool, round collar,
dolman sleeve, sequin covered
bodice.
$100-$150
Courtesy Shirley Friedland

Left:
Detail of fabric

Sweater - c. 1950s
Expressly Hand Decorated for The
May Co. in British Hong Kong
Cream 70% lambs wool, 20% angora
rabbit fur, 10% nylon, sequin bead
bodice and sleeve.
$100-$150

Detail of fabric

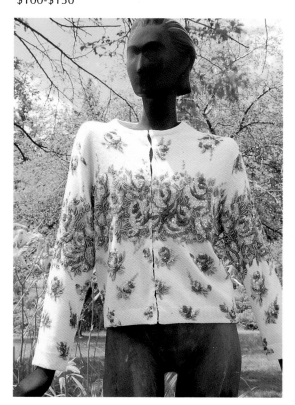

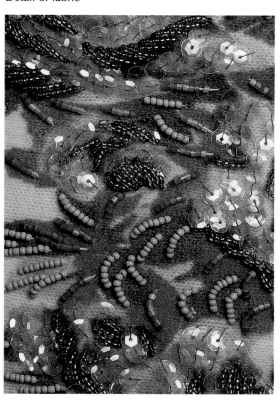

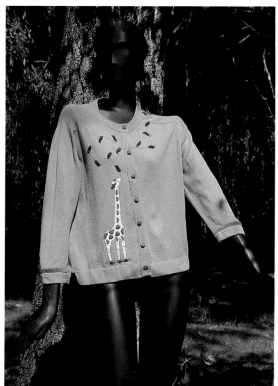

Sweater - c. 1950s
Aqua 100% cashmere, giraffe appliqué.
$50-$75

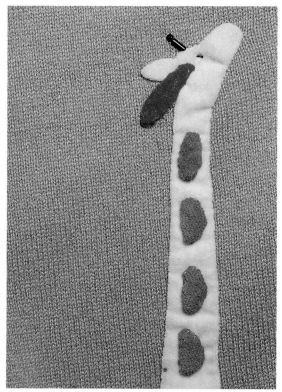

Detail of appliqué

105

Jacket sweater - c. 1950s
Tan 100% pigskin bodice, welt pocket,
and 100% cotton knit long sleeve.
$50-$75

Sweater - c. 1950s
Valentino
Brown 100% cotton bodice,
100% silk polka dot collar.
$75-$100

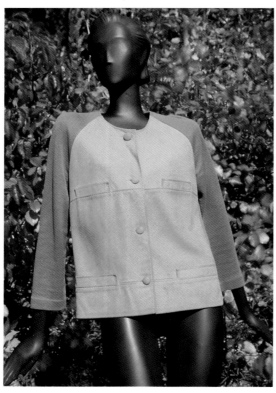 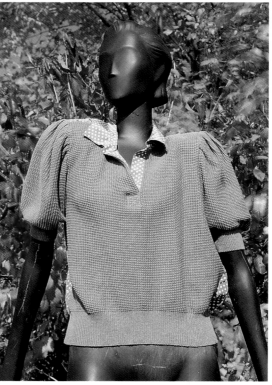

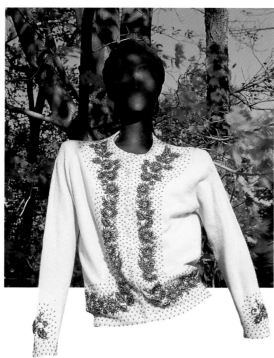 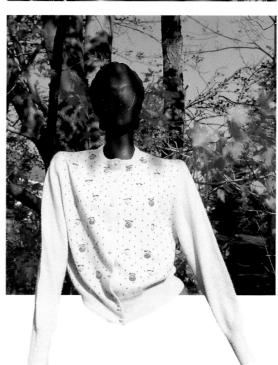

Sweater - c. 1950s
Beige 70% lambs wool, 20% angora, 10%
nylon, beading on front and sleeve.
$40-$60

Sweater - c. 1950s
Beige 100% cashmere
with sea shell beading.
$50-$75

Sweater - c. 1950s
White 100% orlon, beading
on bodice and cuff.
$50-$75

Sweater - c. 1950s
White 100% orlon, sequin
panels, pearl button.
$50-$75

Sweater - c. 1950s
White 100% mohair wool,
rhinestone button.
$40-$60

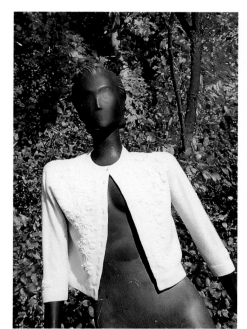

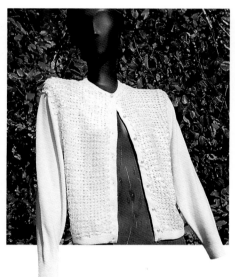

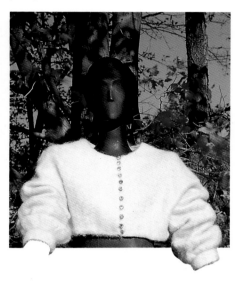

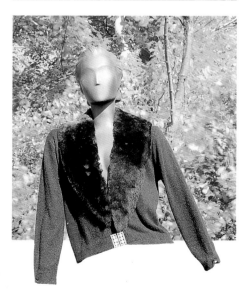

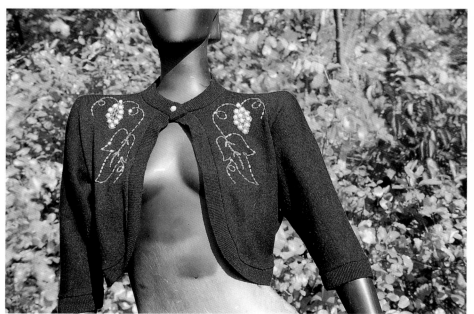

Sweater - c. 1950s
Black 100% orlon acrylic,
mock fur, rhinestone clasp.
$30-$40

Sweater - c. 1950s
Black 100% wool
bolero, beading.
$40-$60

Sweater - c. 1960s
Cream 100% wool,
sequin chevron beading.
$100-$125

Sweater - c. 1960s
Hot pink 100% mohair,
flame stitch.
$40-$60
Courtesy Shirley Friedland

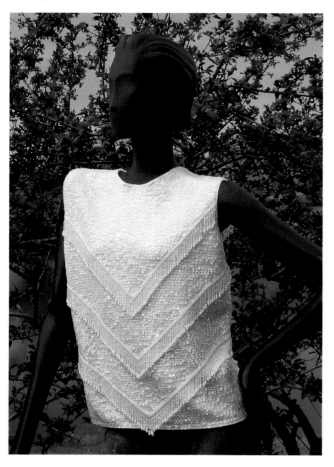

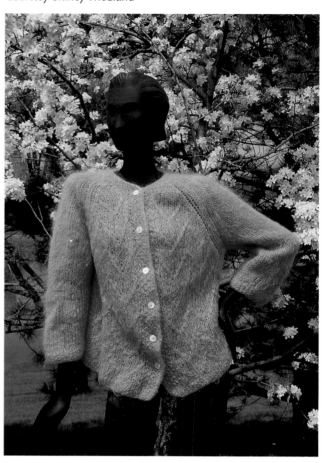

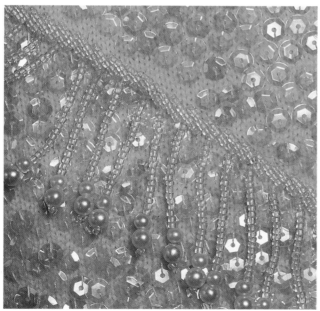

Detail of fabric

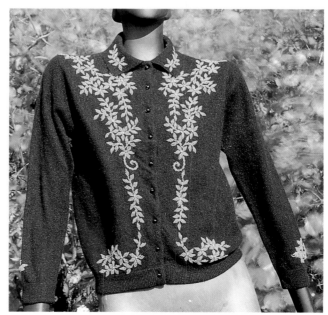

Sweater - c. 1960s
Black 70% lambs wool, 20% angora,
10% nylon, with gold beading.
$50-$75

Sweater - c. 1960s
Apple green 100% mohair,
notched collar, cable stitch.
$35-$50

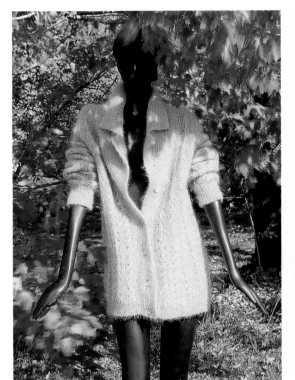

Sweater - c. 1960s
Apple green 100% orlon,
scallop sleeve and edge.
$25-$35

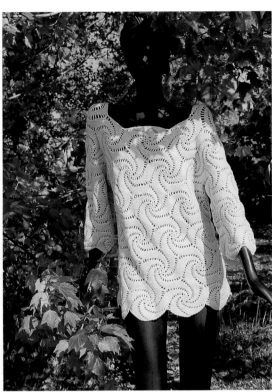

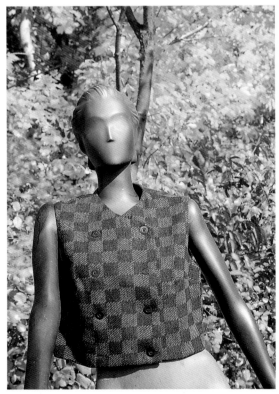

Sweater vest - c. 1960s
Brown 100% wool, double
breasted, sleeveless.
$20-$30

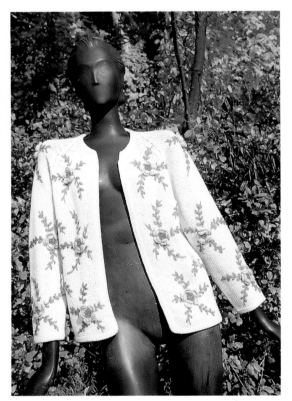

Sweater - c. 1960s
Cream 100% virgin wool,
crochet flower appliqué.
$40-$60

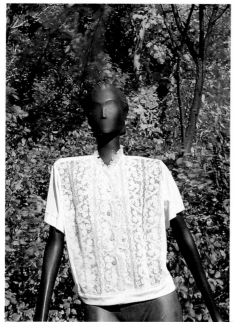

Sweater blouse - c. 1960s
Cream 100% nylon and polyester, short
sleeve, vertical lace panel with ruffle.
$20-$25

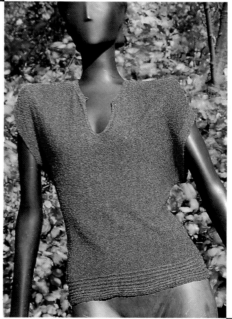

Sweater - c. 1960s
Purple 100% silk, V-neckline.
$30-$40

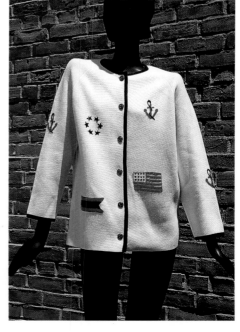

Tennis sweater - c. 1960s
White 100% cotton knit,
nautical motif.
$35-$45
Courtesy Shirley Friedland

Chapter 4
Outerwear

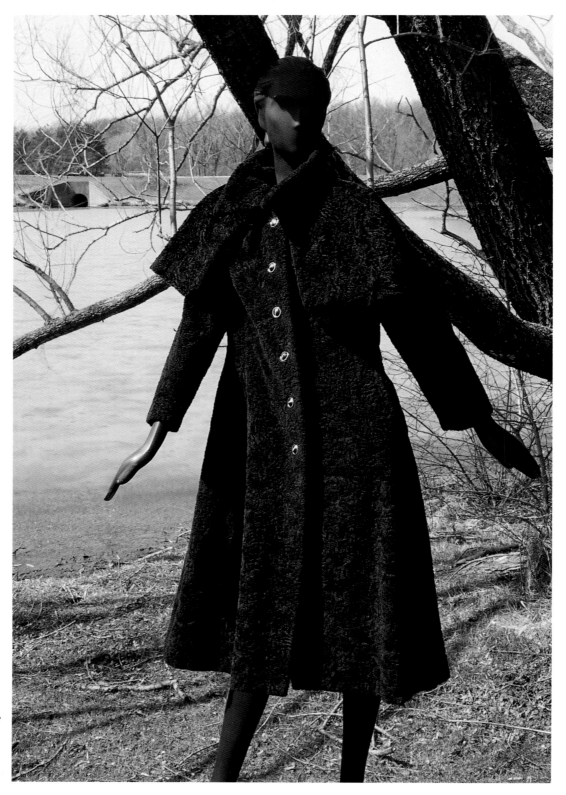

Coat - c. 1950s
Black 100% acrylic,
mock fur cape and
collar.
$50-$75

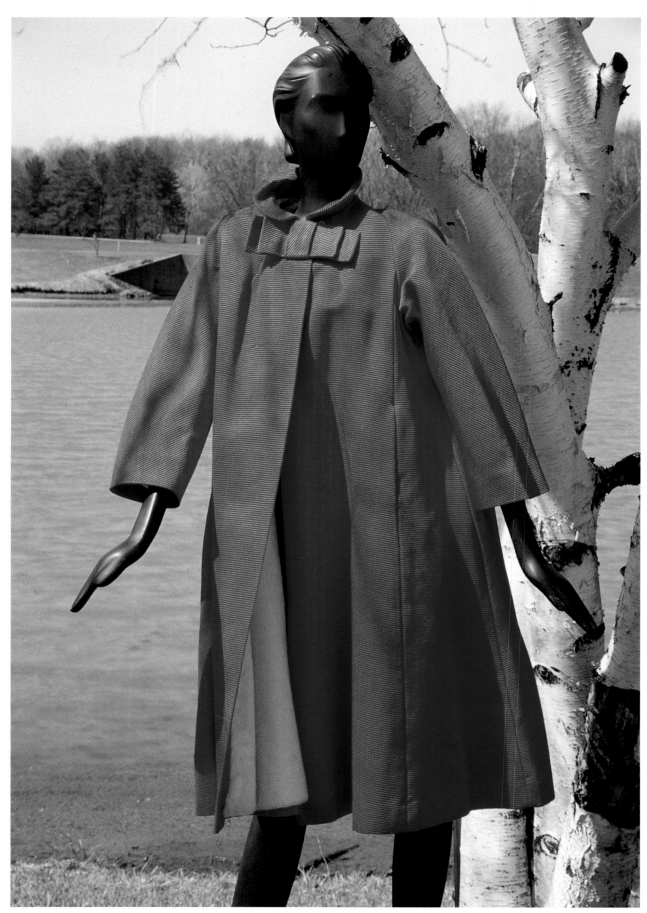

Coat - c. 1950s
The Halle Bros. Co.
Red 100% silk, round collar,
bow, mock fur lining.
$75-$100

112

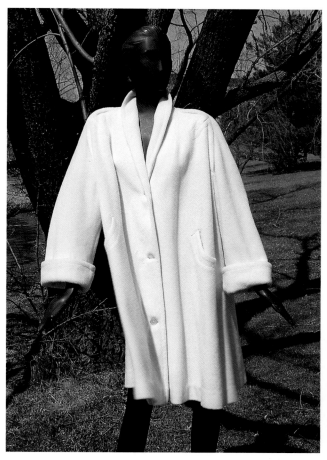

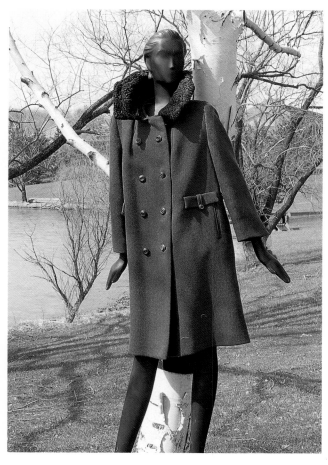

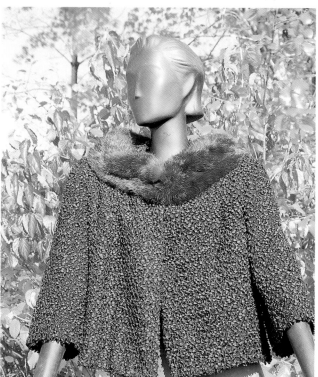

Above left:
Coat - c. 1952
Taylor's, Cleveland
White 100% orlon, first
wash-and-wear coat, shawl
collar.
$50-$75

Above right:
Coat - c. 1950s
Grey 100% polyester knit,
lamb fur collar, double
breasted, flap pocket.
$75-$100

Left:
Jacket - c. 1950s
Black 100% rayon, crochet
ribbon, fur trim.
$60-$80

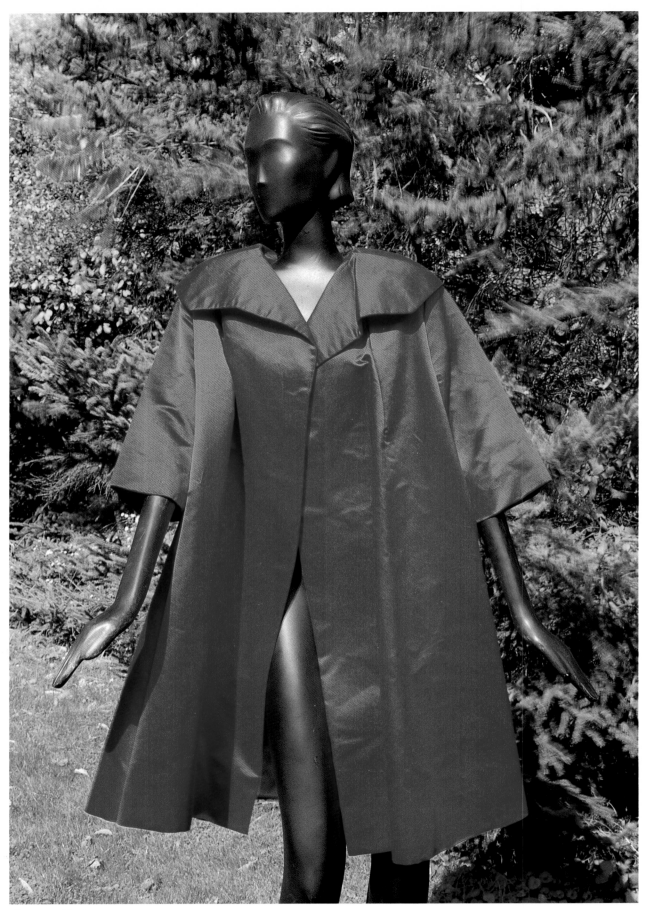

Coat - c. 1950s
Saks Fifth Avenue
Hot pink 100% silk, square collar, 3/4 sleeve.
$75-$100
Courtesy Studio Moderne

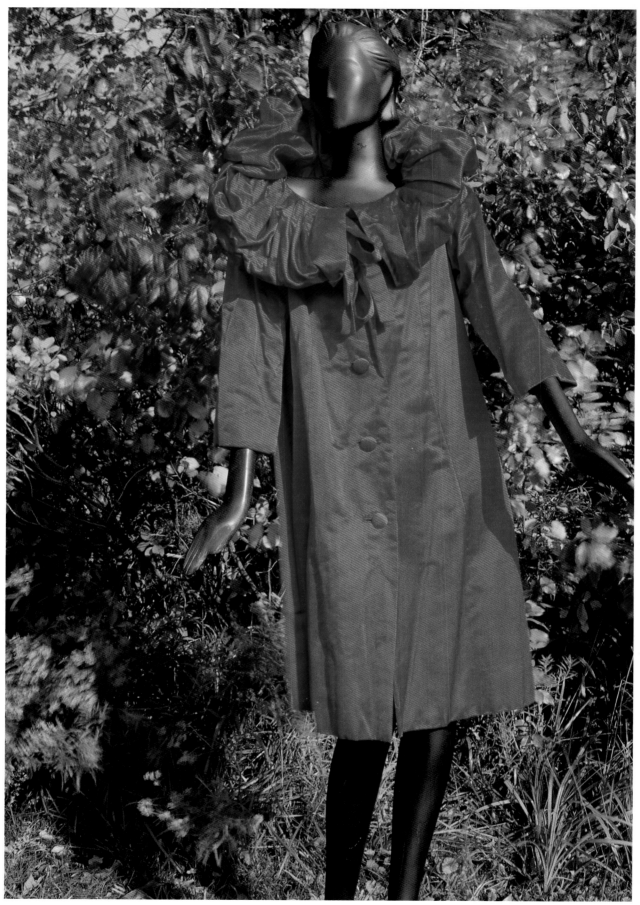

Coat - c. 1950s
Sylvan Rich for Martini
Hot pink 100% silk, 3/4 sleeve, bubble collar.
$100-$150

Coat - c. 1969
Navy 100% wool, notched collar,
double breasted, red lining.
$50-$75

Coat - c. 1962
Halle Bros. Co.
Red 100% wool, notched
collar, large brass button.
$50-$75

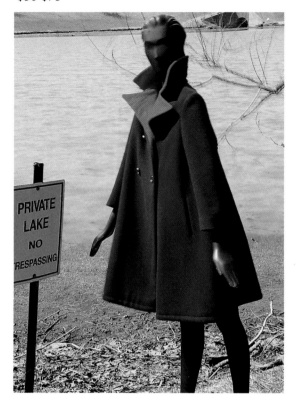

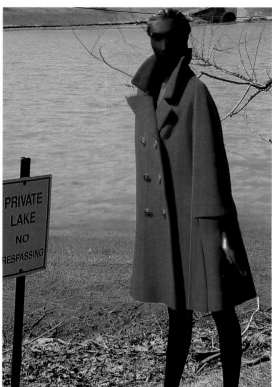

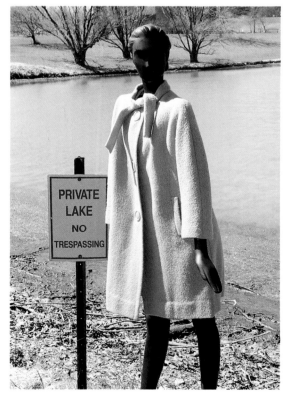

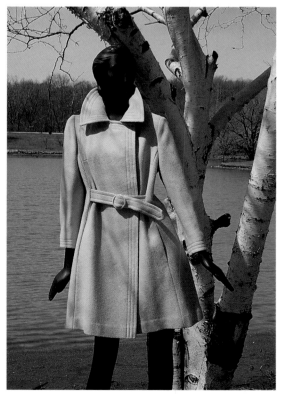

Coat - c. 1960s
White 100% wool.
$50-$75

Coat - c. 1960s
Beige 100% wool, top
stitched, belted.
$50-$75

Coat - c. 1960s
Black 100% wool, mink
collar, cuff, crochet button.
$100-$150

Detail of button

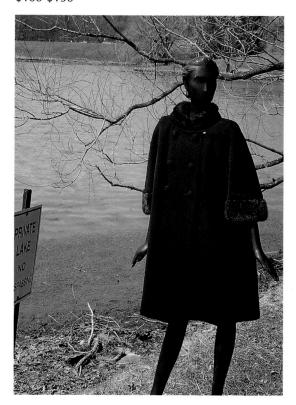

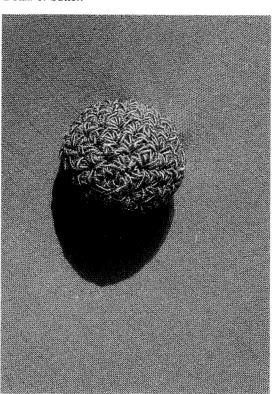

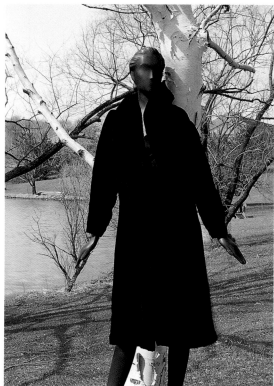

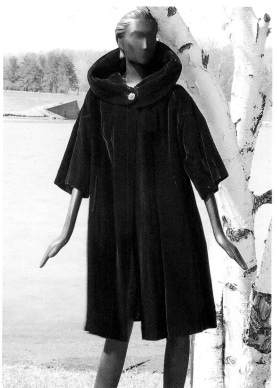

Coat - c. 1960s
Black velvet with shawl collar.
$75-$100

Coat - c. 1960s
Deep blue velvet, rhinestone closure.
$75-$100

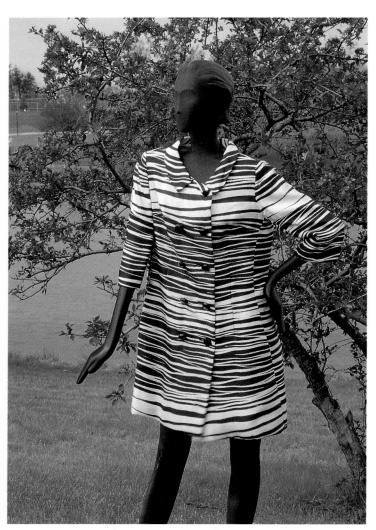

Coat - c. 1960s
Henry Harris, Cincinnati
Zebra print 100% silk, double breasted.
$75-$100

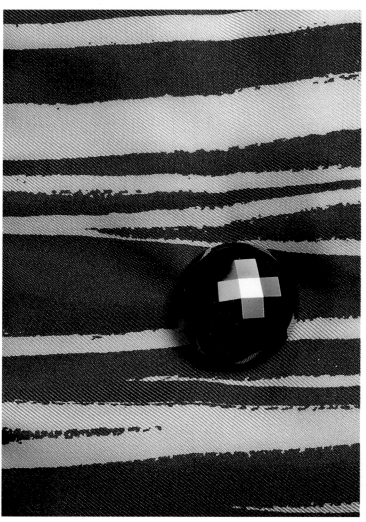

Detail of fabric

Label

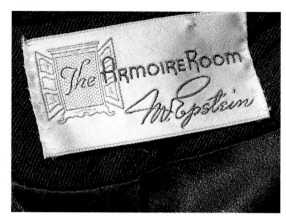

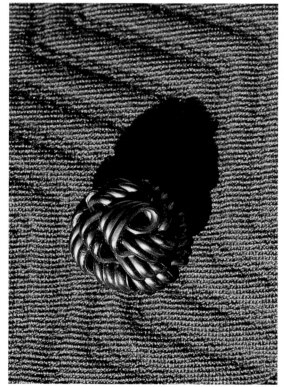

Detail of button

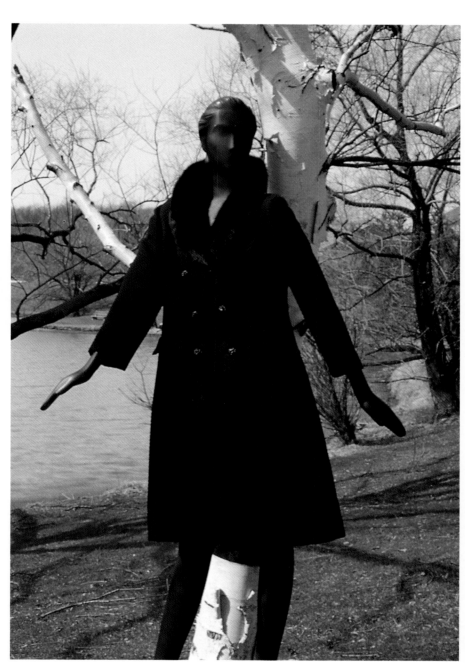

Coat - c. 1960s
Armoire Room
Black 100% cotton, twill weave,
mink collar, plastic button.
$100-$150

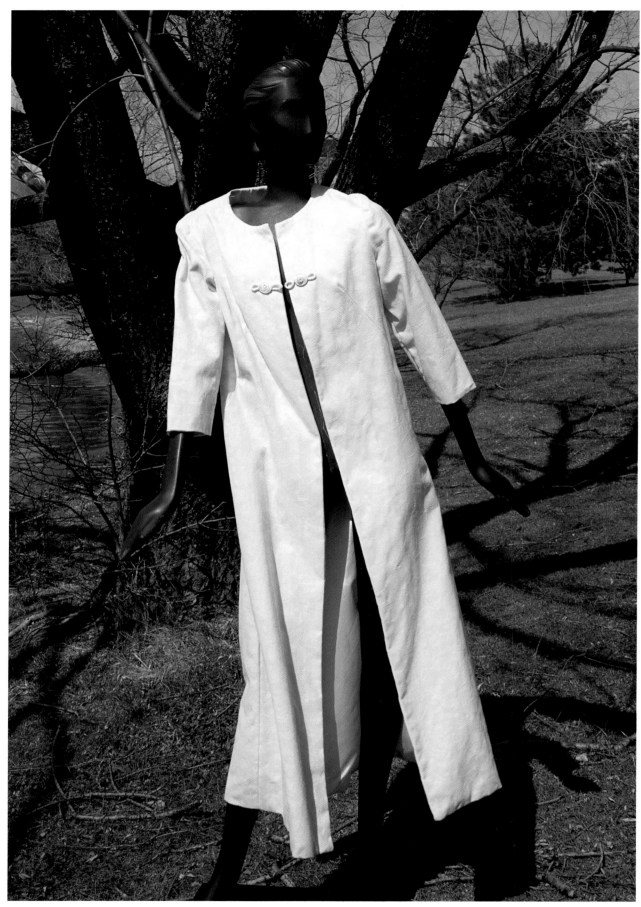

Coat - c. 1960s
Cream 100% cotton, round
neckline, frog closure.
$50-$75

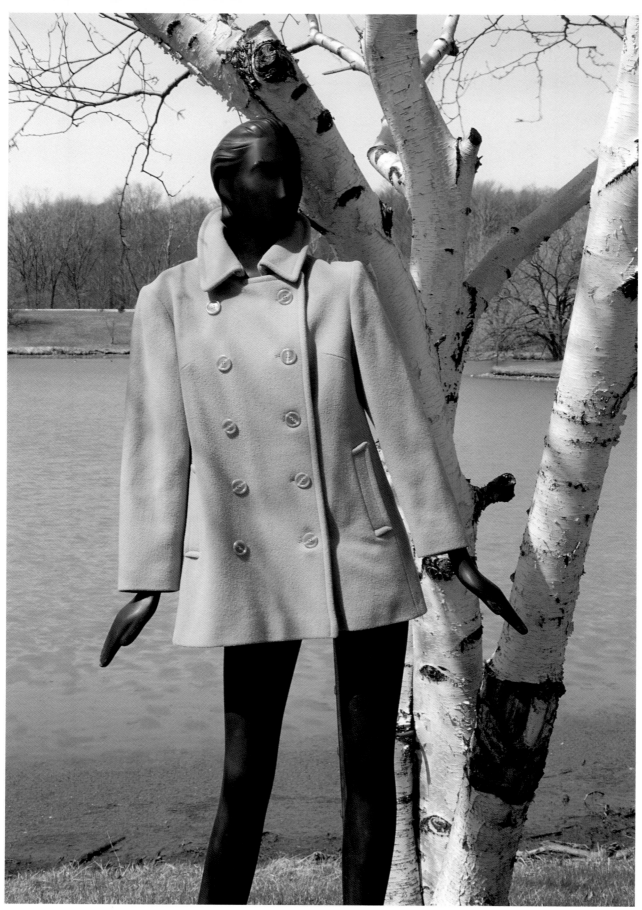

Coat - c. 1960s
Tan 100% wool, double breasted.
$50-$75

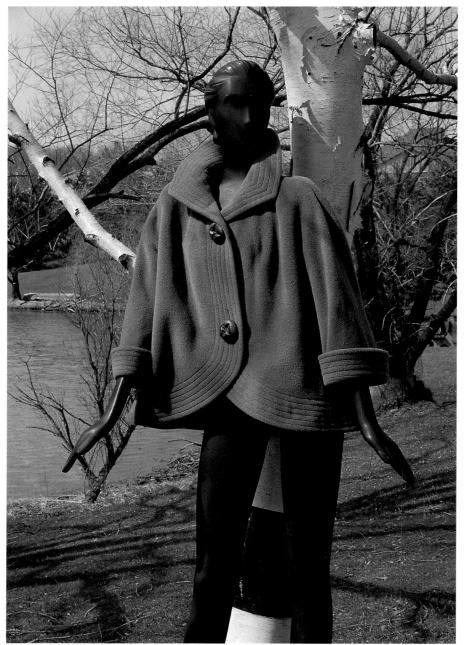

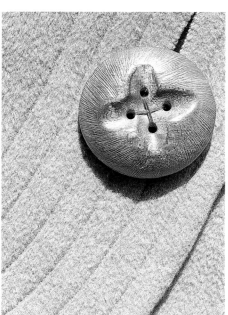

Above:
Jacket - c. 1960
Pattullo — Jo Copeland
Tan 100% wool, top stitched
collar, cuff, wooden button.
$50-$75

Left:
Detail of button

Jacket - c. 1960s
Saks Fifth Avenue
White 100% silk, crochet ribbon
fabric, round neckline, long sleeve.
$75-$100

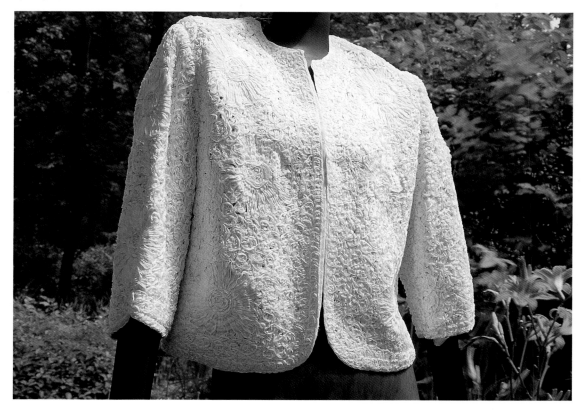

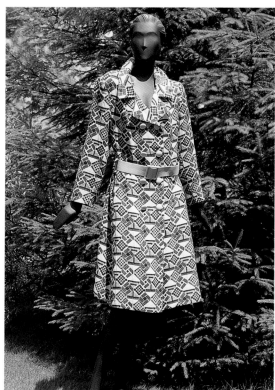

Coat - c. 1960s
Printzess Fashion, Halle Bros. Co.
Multi 100% cotton, geometric bold
print, notched collar, leather belt.
$60-$80

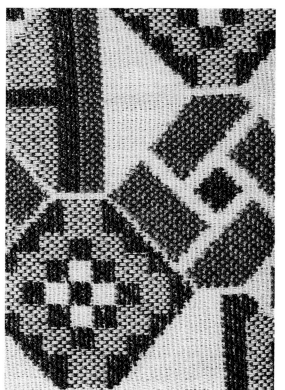

Detail of fabric

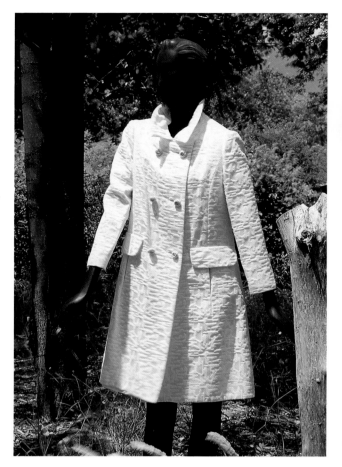

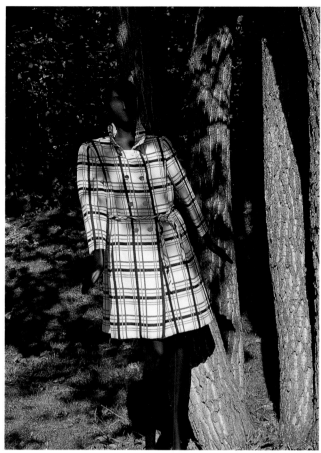

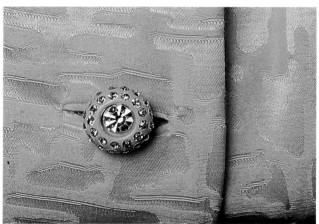

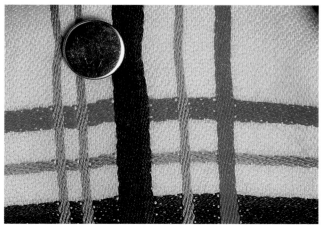

Top left:
Coat - c. 1960s
Yellow 100% silk, collar, long sleeve, double breasted, rhinestone button, flap pocket.
$50-$75

Lower left:
Detail of button

Top right:
Coat - c. 1960s
Lillie Rubin
Multi-plaid 100% wool, double breasted, brass button.
$75-$100

Center right:
Label

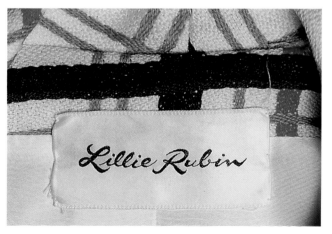

Detail of fabric

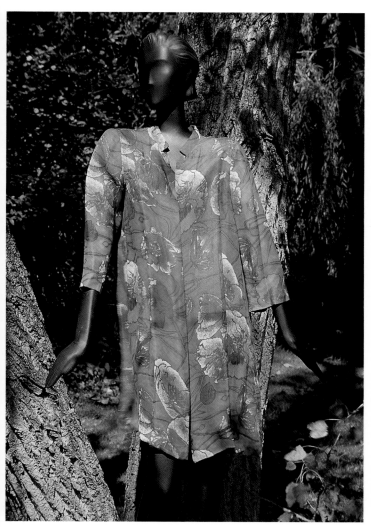

Coat - c. 1960s
Green 100% silk, floral print.
$60-$80

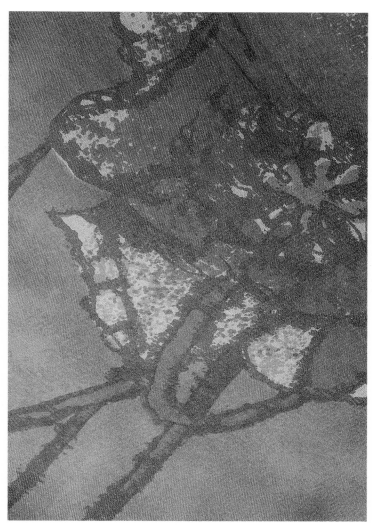

Detail of fabric

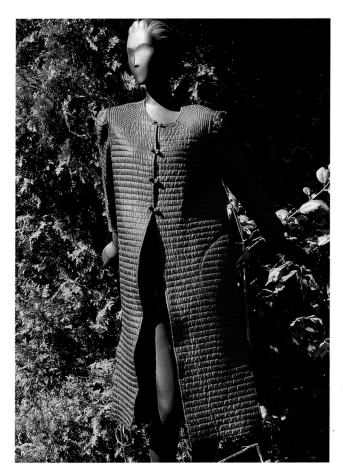

Top:
Label

Bottom:
Jacket - c. 1960s
Geoffrey Beene
Cream 100% wool,
notched collar, braid
trim.
$75-$125

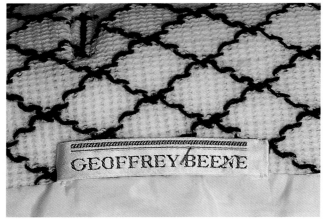

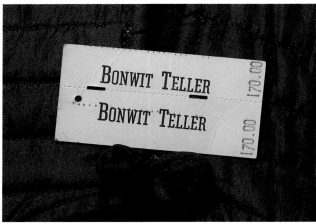

Top:
Coat - c. 1965
Bonwit Teller
Purple 100% silk, reversible,
quilted, frog closure.
$100-$150

Bottom:
Label (original tag)

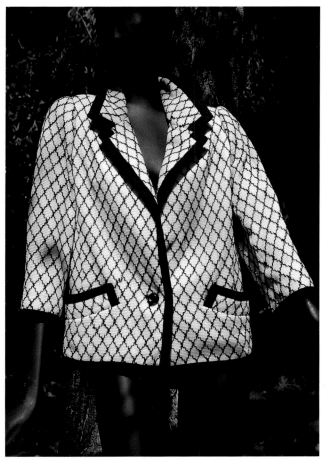

Bottom:
Jacket - c. 1960s
Modelia — Shandra
Black mock fur, woven pile,
notched collar, flap pocket.
$50-$75

Top:
Label

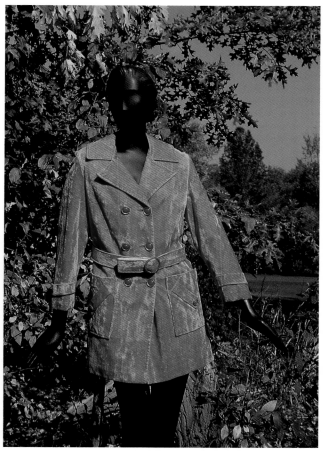

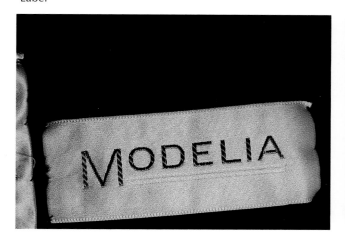

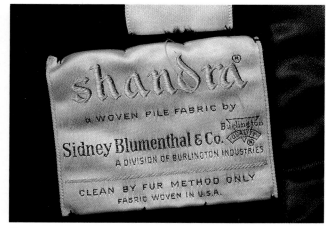

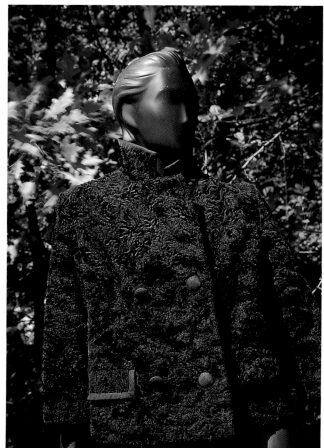

Top:
Jacket - c. 1960s
Trail Tracer
Orange 100% suede velour, notched
collar, double breasted, belted.
$50-$75
Courtesy Studio Moderne

Bottom:
Label

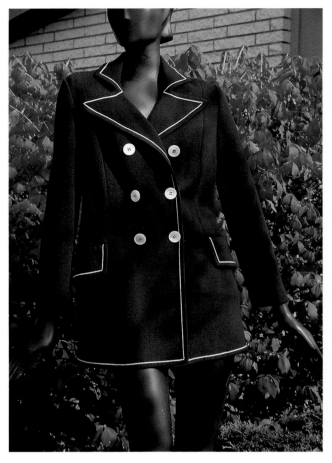

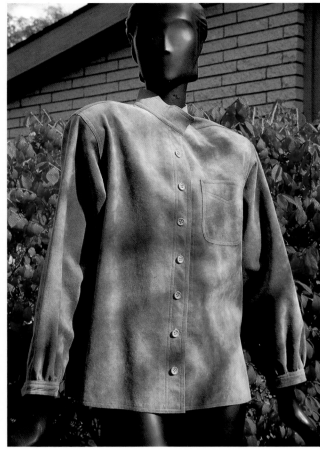

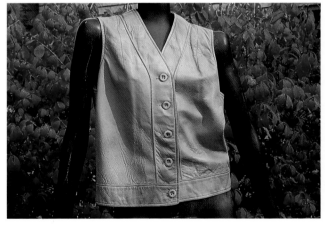

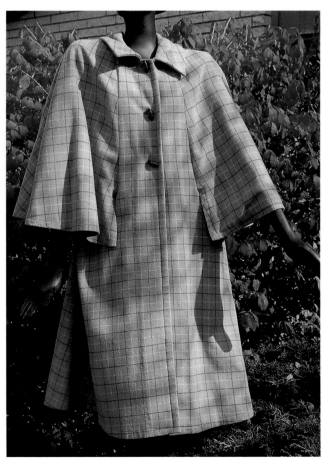

Top left:
Jacket - c. 1969
Gino Paoli, Italy
Navy 100% wool, notched
collar, white braid, double
breasted, flap pocket.
$75-$100
Courtesy Shirley Friedland

Top right:
Jacket - c. 1960
Blassport
Khaki green Skinner ultra
suede, long sleeve, banded
cuff.
$60-$80
Courtesy Shirley Friedland

Bottom left:
Vest - c. 1960s
Tan leather, V-neckline,
sleeveless.
$40-$60
Courtesy Shirley Friedland

Bottom right:
Coat - c. 1960s
Plaid 100% wool, spring
weight, cape sleeve.
$75-$100
Courtesy Shirley Friedland

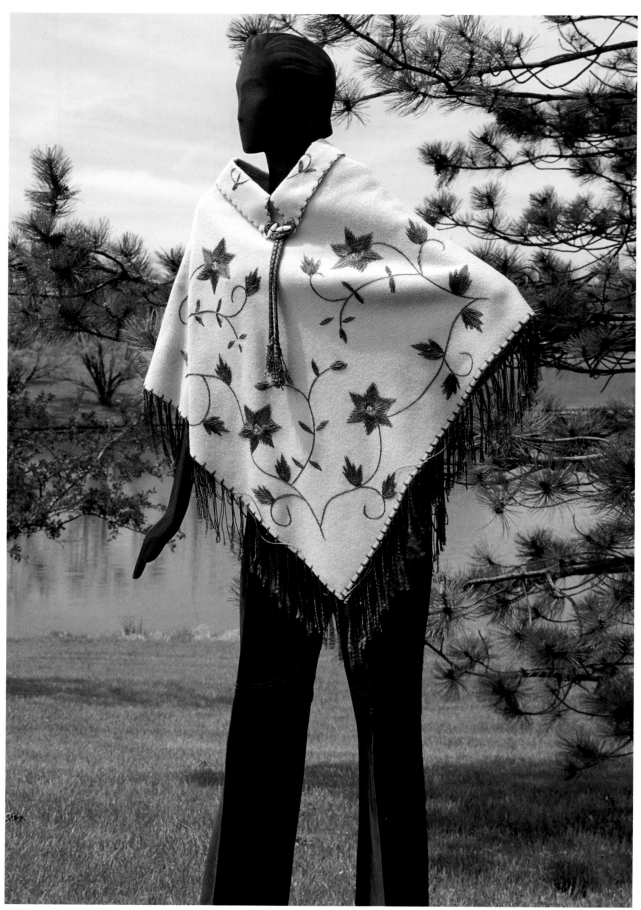

Poncho - c. 1966
Tan 100% wool, embroidery, fringe.
$50-$75

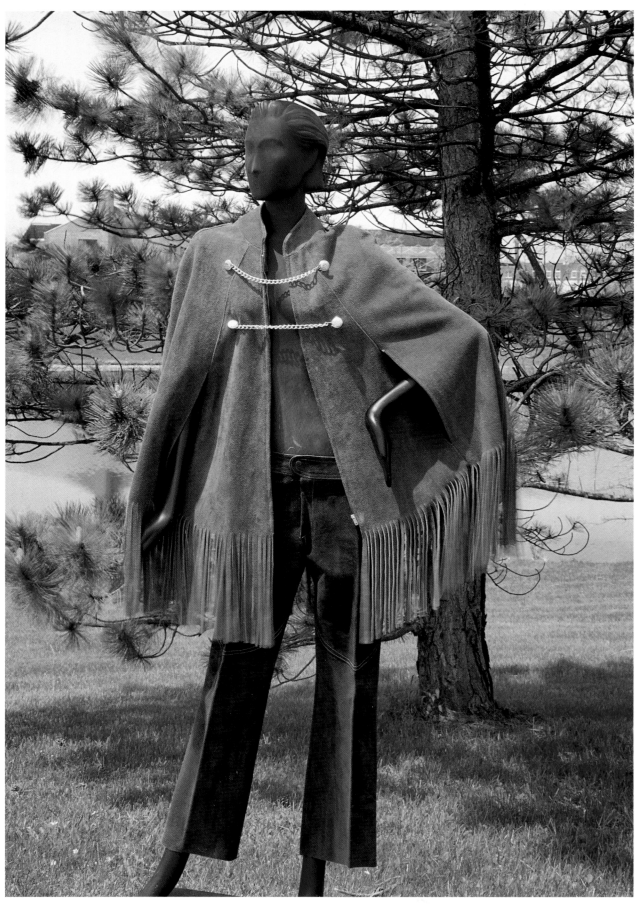

Cape and pant - c. 1969
Canada
Brown suede, slit opening, fringe
and matching pant with flared leg.
$150-$175

130   *Courtesy Shirley Friedland*

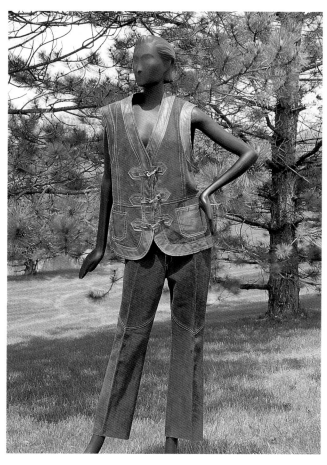

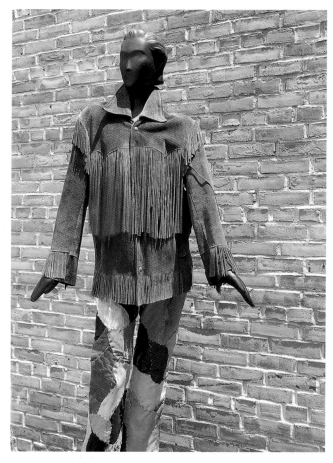

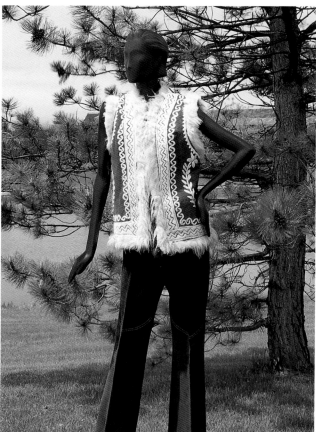

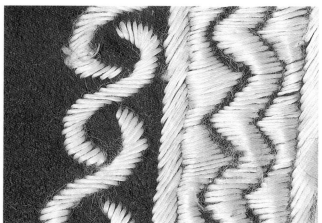

Top left:
Vest - c. 1965
Brown suede with leather
trim, metal closure.
$50-$75

Left:
Vest - c. 1965
Brown suede, embroidery,
fur lined.
$70-$90

Top right:
Jacket - c. 1968
Purple suede, collar, long
sleeve, fringe bodice, cuff,
zipper closure and leather.
$100-$125
Author

Above:
Detail of embroidery

131

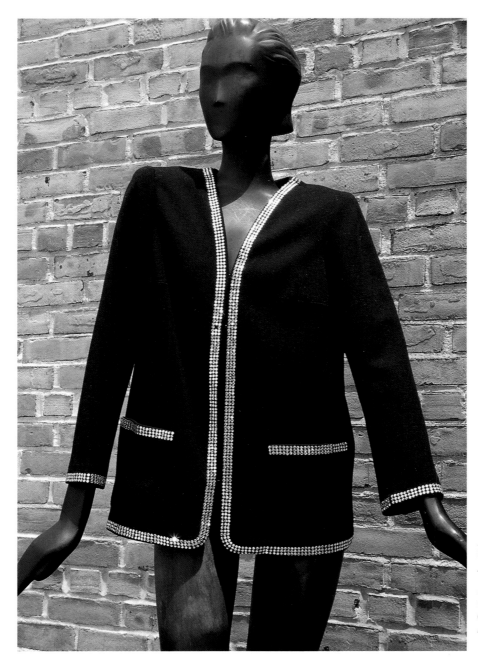

Jacket - c. 1960s
Shannon Rodgers for
Jerry Silverman
Black 100% wool,
rhinestone trim.
$175-$200
*Courtesy Shirley
Friedland*

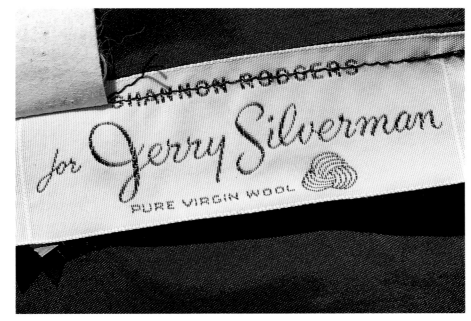

Label

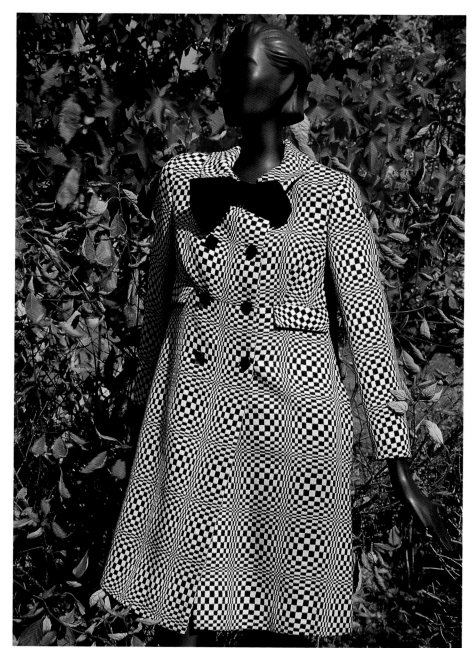

Coat - c. 1960s
Mansfield Original by
Frank Russell, Made in
England
Op Art print 100% wool,
bow, collar, double
breasted.
$100-$150
Courtesy Studio Moderne

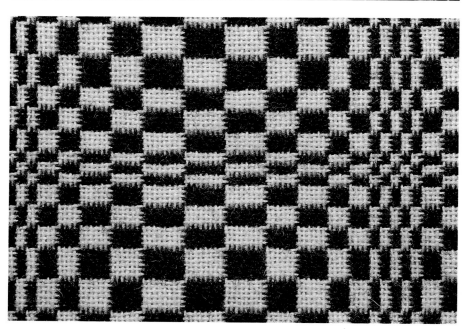

Detail of fabric

Next page:
Detail of fabric

133

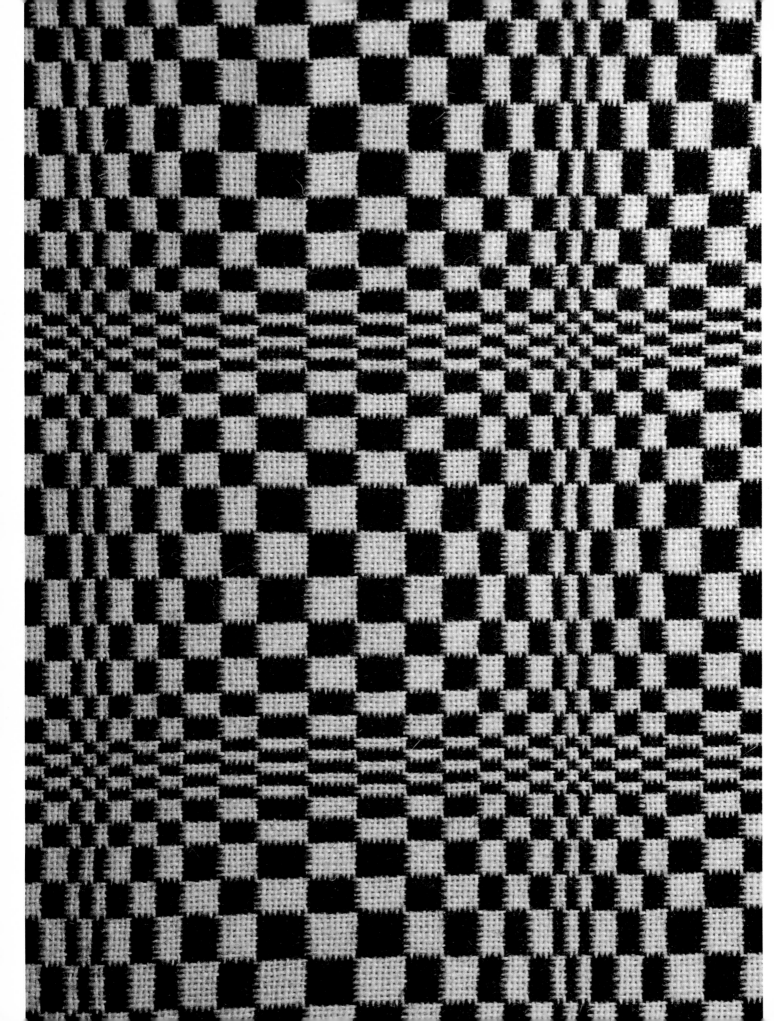

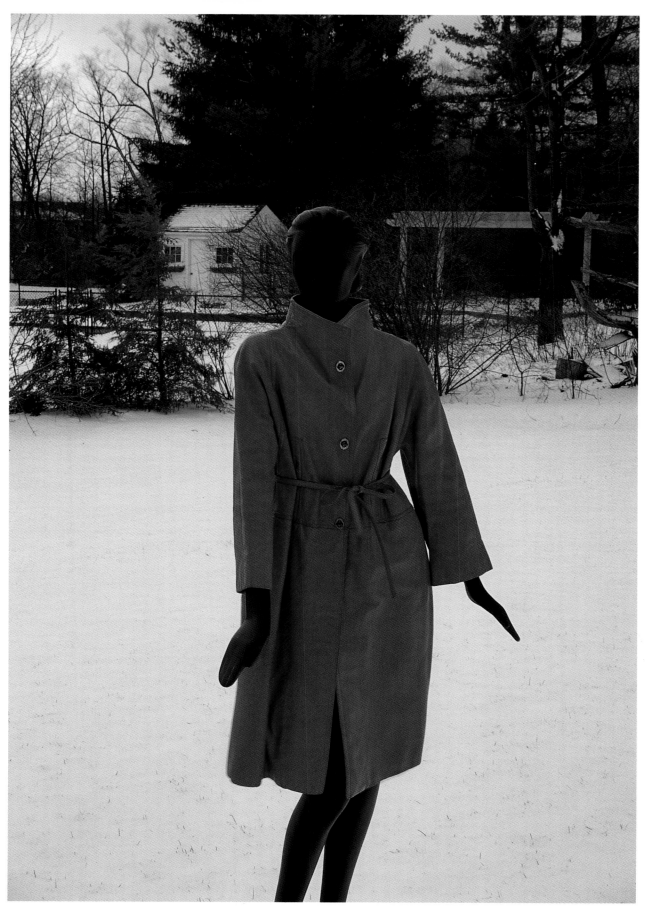

Coat - c. 1960s
Bonnie Cashin
Rust-orange leather, standing collar, belted.
$100-$150
Courtesy Shirley Friedland

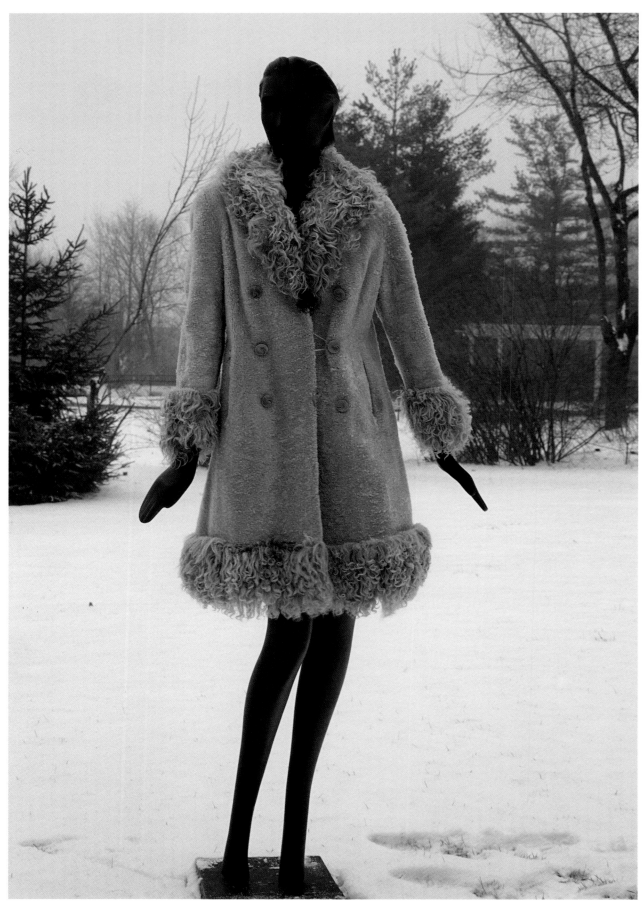

Coat - c. 1960s
Cream sheared lamb, double breasted,
Tibetan lamb collar, cuff, hem.
$100-$150
Courtesy Shirley Friedland

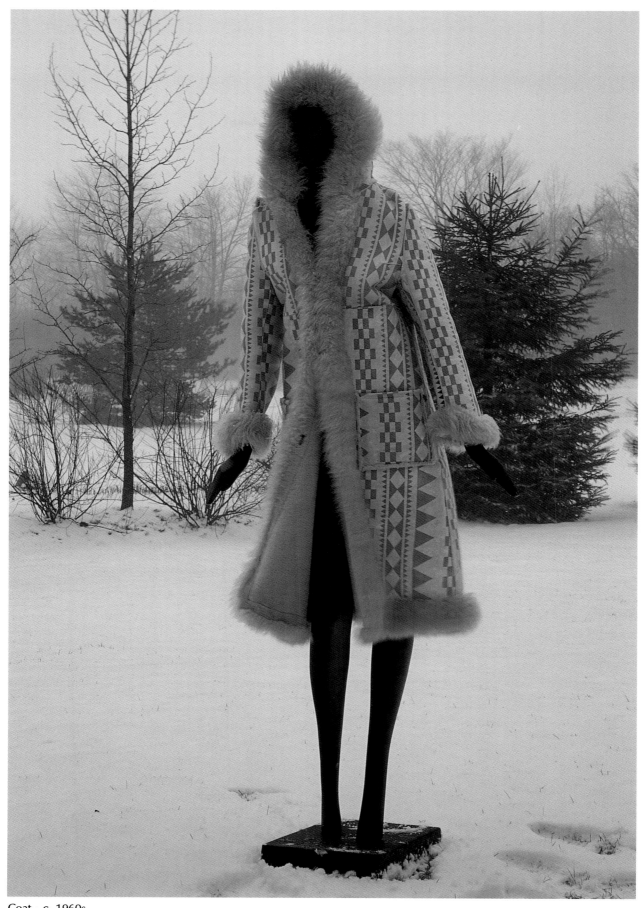

Coat - c. 1960s
Cream shearling, stenciled geometric
motif, lamb trim hood, cuff, hem.
$150-$175
Author

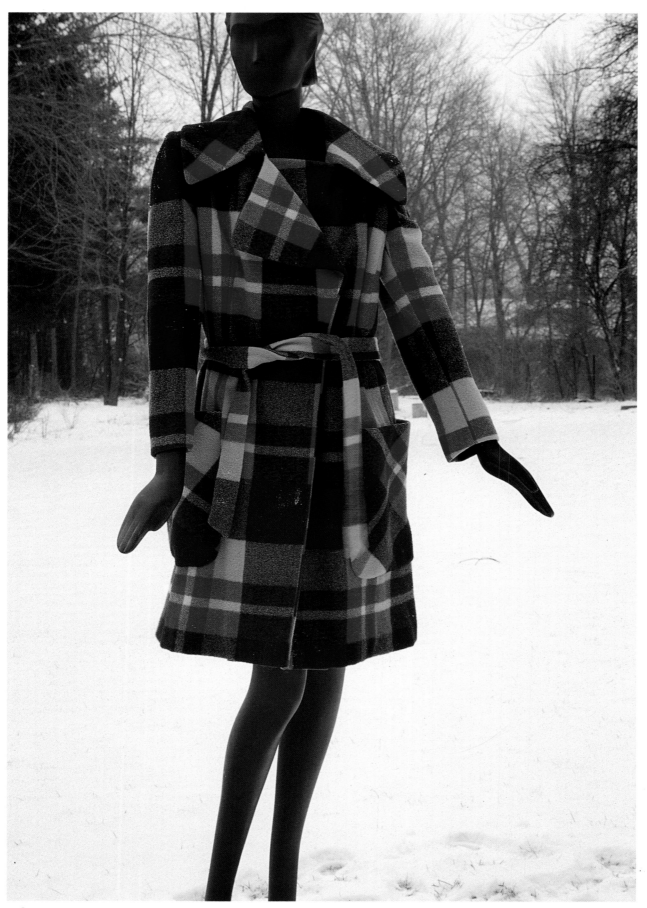

Coat - c. 1960s
Multi-plaid 100% wool, notched
collar, patch pocket, belted.
$75-$125

Courtesy Shirley Friedland

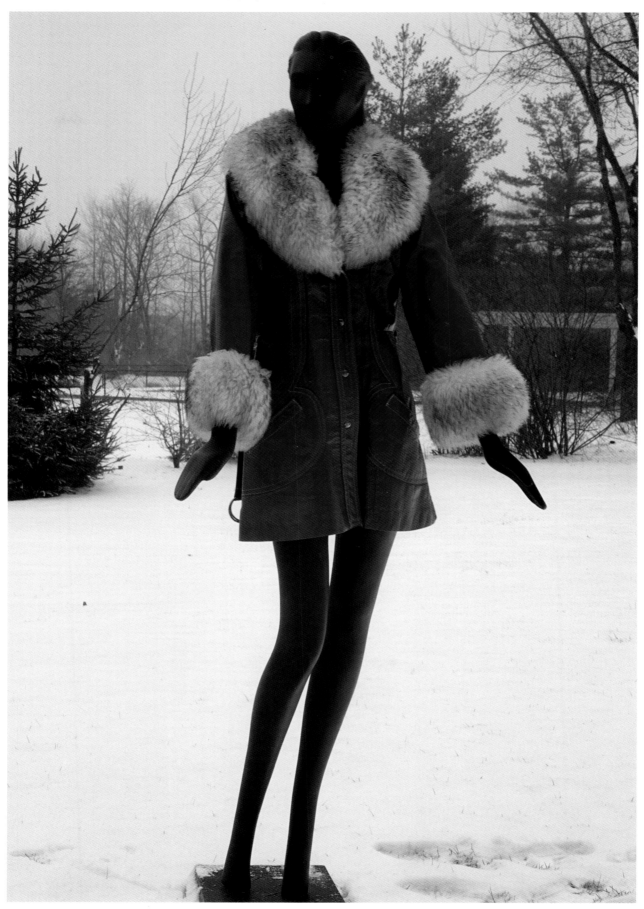

Coat - c. 1960s
Toast leather, patch pocket,
lamb collar, cuff.
$75-$100
Courtesy Shirley Friedland

Chapter 5

Casual/Hostess

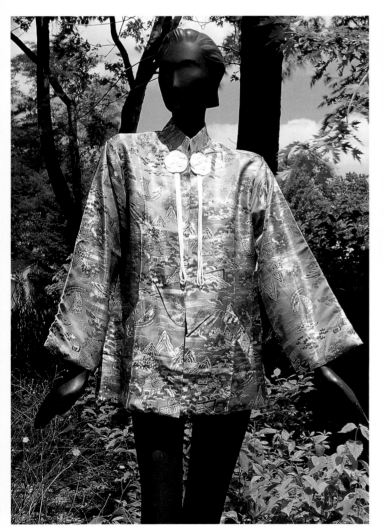

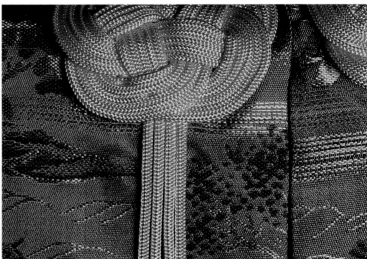

Left:
Oriental tunic - c. 1950s
Turquoise 100% silk, mandarin collar,
long sleeve, pocket, braided knot
closure.
$50-$75

Above:
Detail

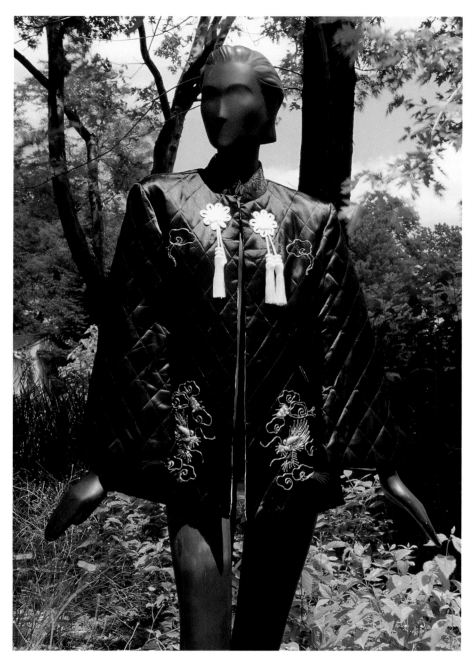

Jacket - c. 1950s
Black 100% silk, quilted
mandarin collar, gold
embroidery, white tassel
closure.
$50-$75

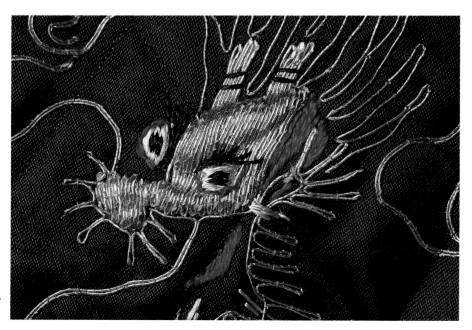

Detail of embroidery

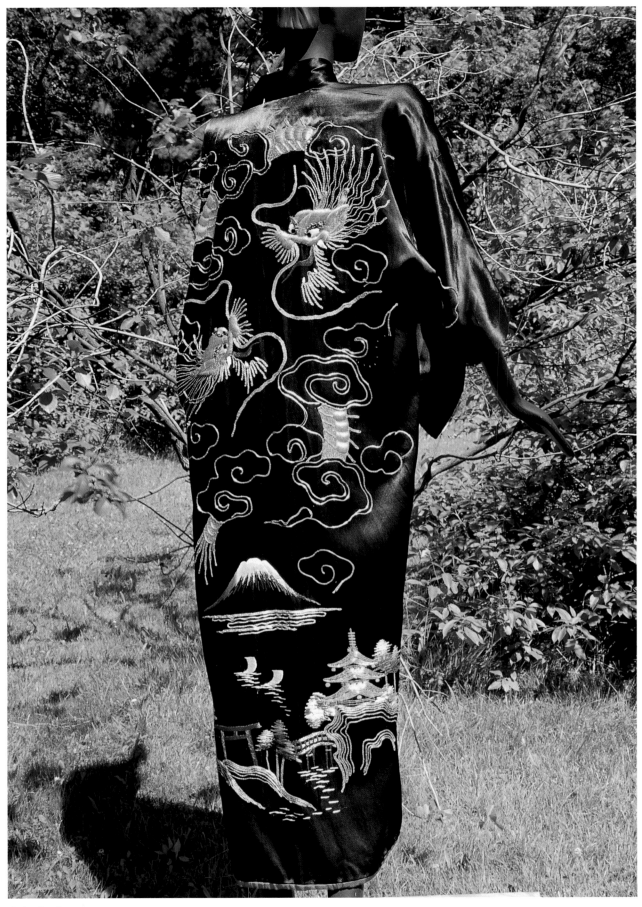

Robe back

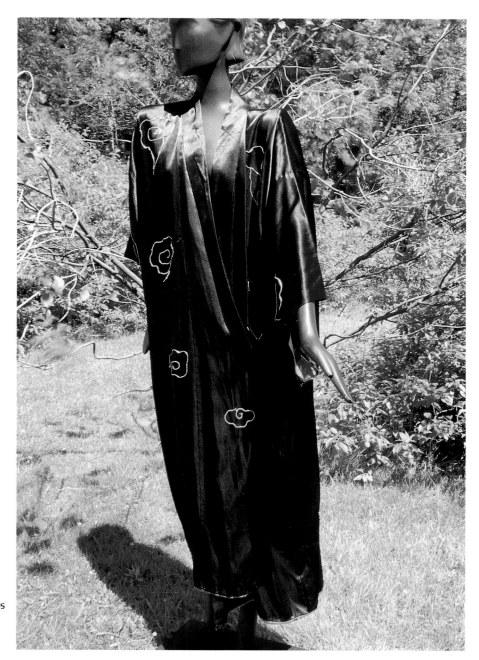

Kimono robe - c. 1950s
Black 100% silk, with
gold embroidery.
$100-$125

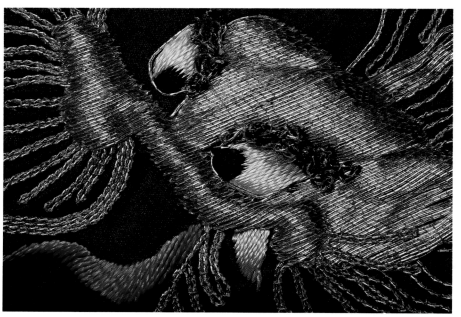

Detail of embroidery

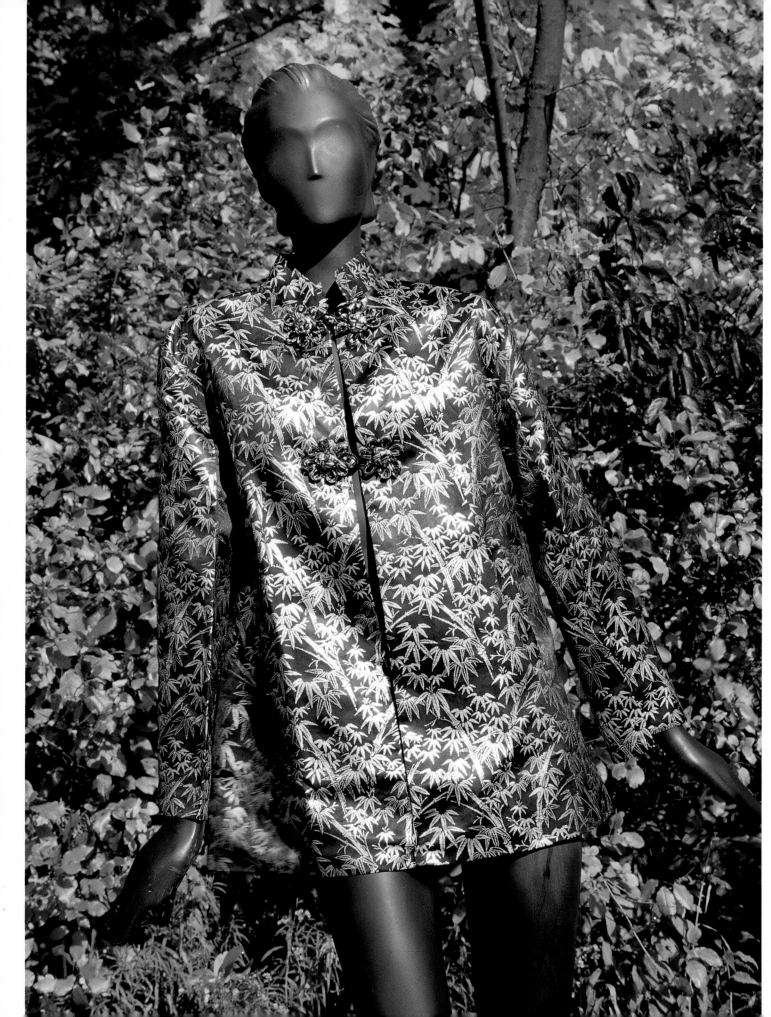

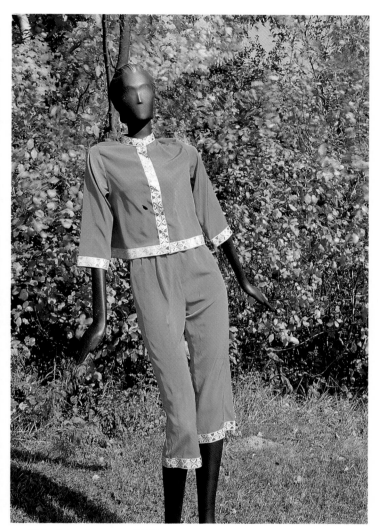

Oriental pajama - c. 1950s
Aqua 100% silk, metallic ribbon trim.
$40-$60

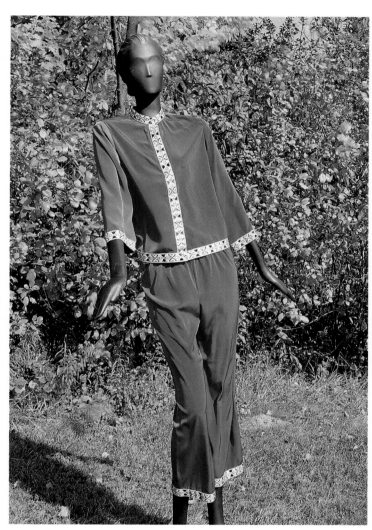

Oriental pajama - c. 1950s
Royal blue 100% silk, metallic ribbon trim.
$40-$60

Opposite:
Oriental tunic - c. 1950s
Black 100% silk, frog closure.
$50-$75

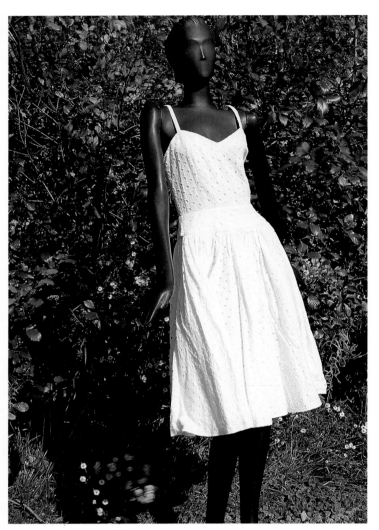

Sun dress - c. 1950s
White 100% cotton,
sweetheart neckline,
gathered skirt.
$25-$35

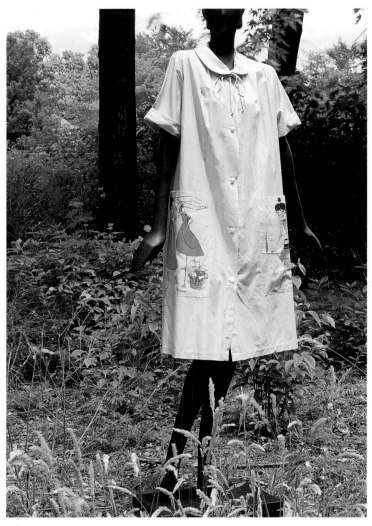

Above:
House coat - c. 1959
Theo
Beige 100% cotton,
round collar, short
sleeve, patch pocket.
$25-$35

Right:
Detail of pocket

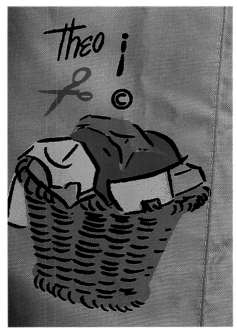

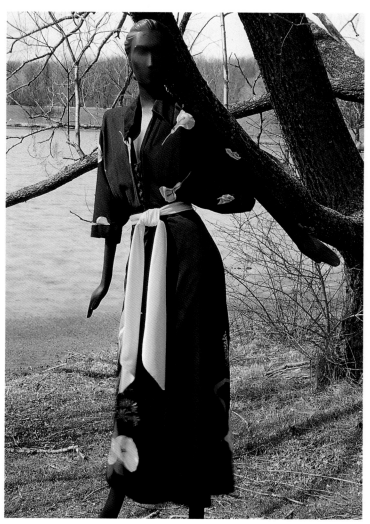

Hostess dress - c. 1960s
Saks Fifth Avenue, Made in England
Black 100% silk, lily motif, yellow sash.
$50-$75

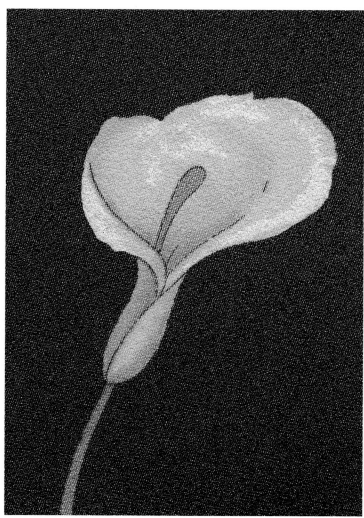

Detail of fabric

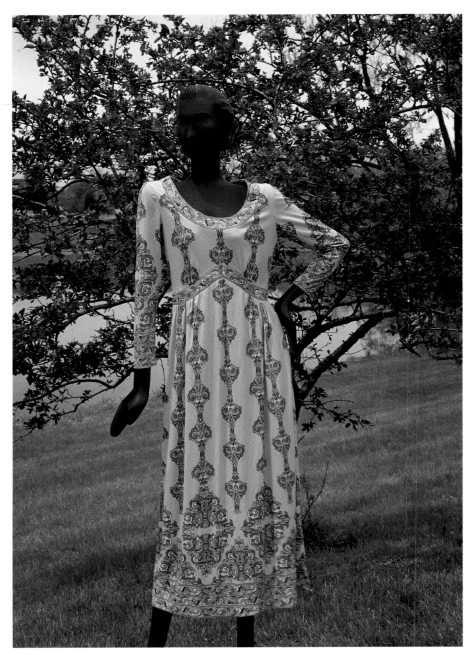

Hostess dress - c. 1960s
Maurice
Aqua 100% polyester
print, scoop neckline,
long sleeve.
$50-$75

Detail of fabric

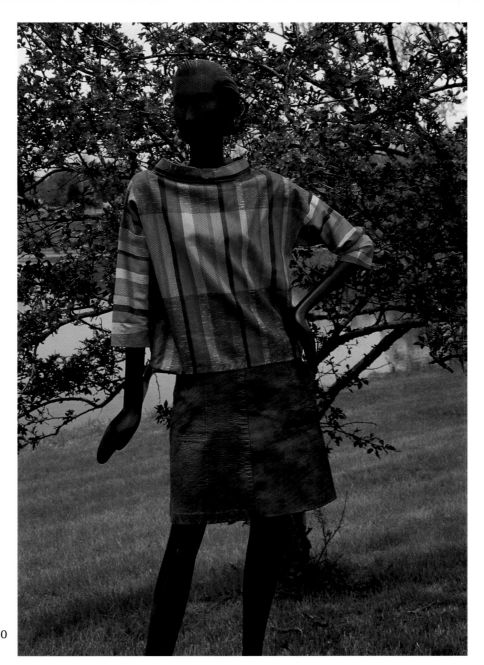

Top and skirt - c. 1965
Multi-stripe 100% Botany
wool top, designed by
Shirley Friedland; leather
mini skirt.
Top $50-$75; skirt $30-$50
Courtesy Shirley Friedland

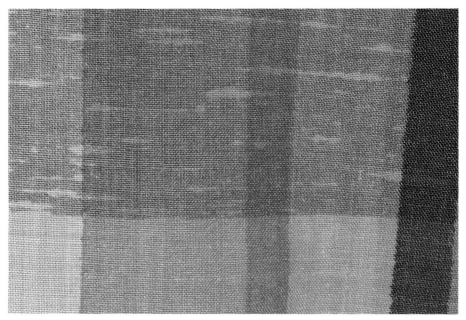

Detail of fabric

Sun dress - c. 1960s
Lilly Pulitzer Inc.
Aqua 100% cotton floral
print, beaded collar.
$50-$75

Hostess dress - c. 1960s
Multi-floral 100% cotton
bold print, ruffle skirt.
$50-$75

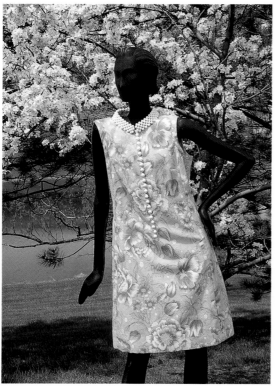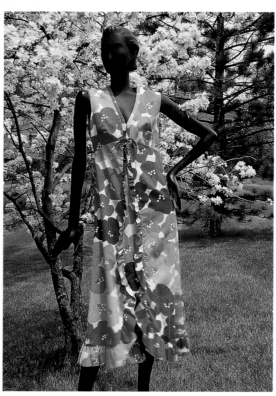

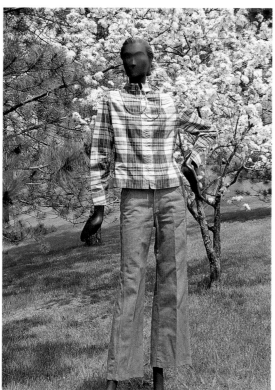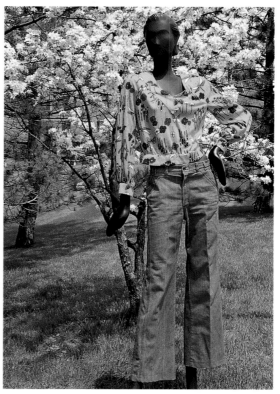

Top and jeans - c. 1969
Top 100% cotton plaid, designed by
Shirley Friedland; Wrangler jeans 100%
denim with red trim, flared leg.
$40-$60
Courtesy Shirley Friedland

Top and jeans - c. 1960s
Polyester yellow print top, designed by
Shirley Friedland; Wrangler jeans 100%
denim with red trim, flared leg.
$40-$60
Courtesy Shirley Friedland

Blouse - c. 1960s
Light green cotton, Mexican embroidery
appliqué, elastic sleeve, designed by
Shirley Friedland.
$50-$75
Courtesy Shirley Friedland

Detail of embroidery

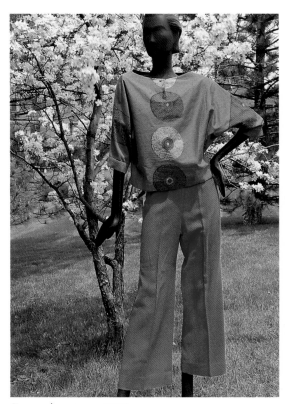

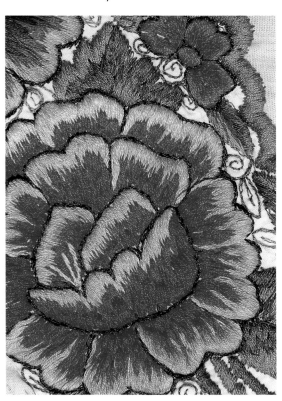

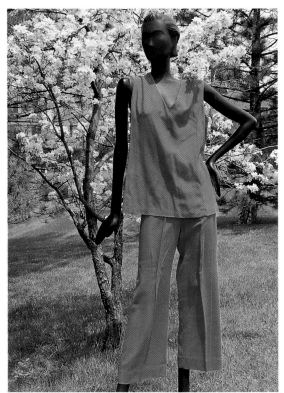

Top and pant - c. 1969
Top 100% cotton green print
and pant 100% silk flared leg.
$50-$75
Courtesy Shirley Friedland

Top and pant - c. 1960s
Top 100% silk, V-neckline, sleeveless
and matching pant with flared leg,
designed by Shirley Friedland.
$60-$80
Courtesy Shirley Friedland

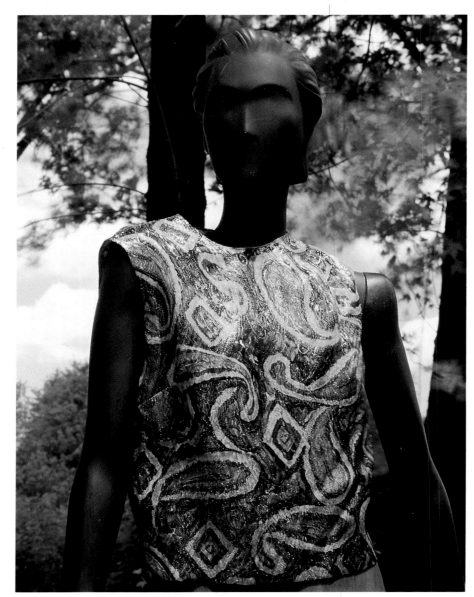

Top - c. 1960s
Malbe Original
Green 100% silk, bold
metallic paisley print,
round neckline,
sleeveless.
$40-$60

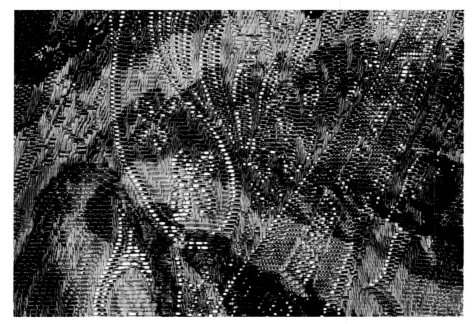

Detail of fabric

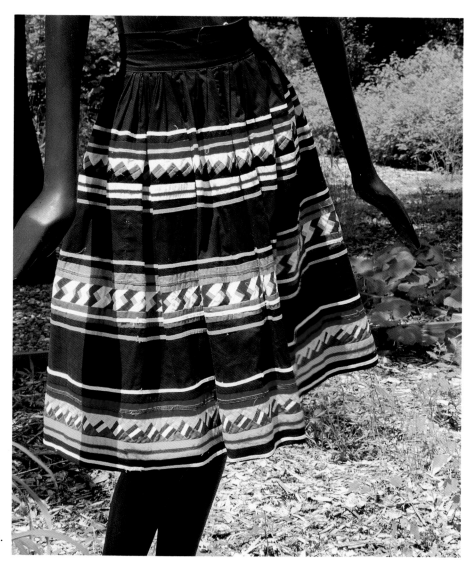

Skirt - c. 1960s
Navy 100% cotton,
appliqué bands, multi-
color, gathered waistline.
$75-$100

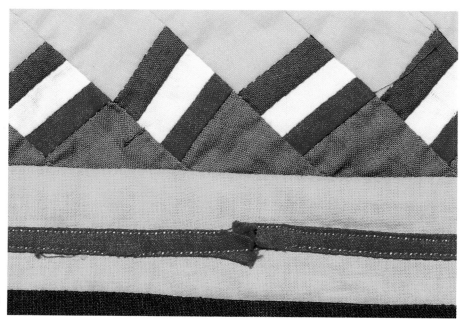

Detail of fabric

153

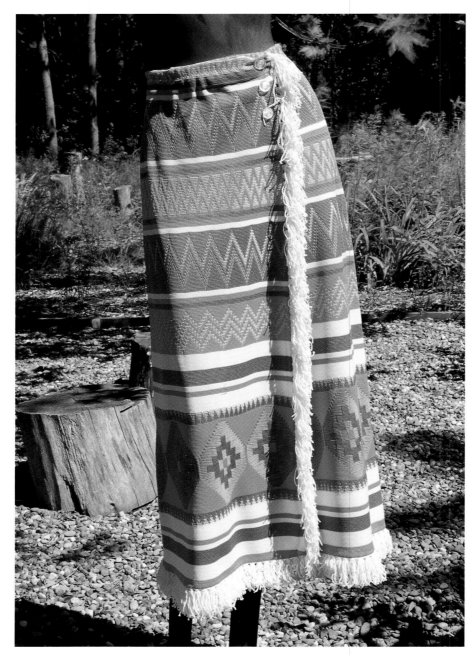

Skirt - c. 1960s
Multi 100% polyester knit,
bold geometric print, elastic
waistline, wrap, fringe trim,
button closure.
$40-$60
*Courtesy Sandra Burdette
Mills*

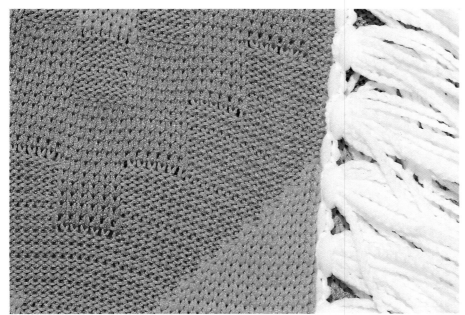

Detail of fabric

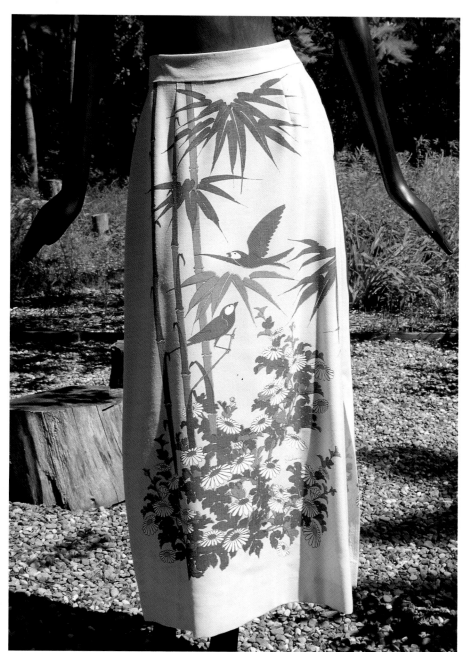

Skirt - c. 1960s
Shaheen
Pink 100% linen print,
zipper closure, side kick slit.
$40-$60
Courtesy Sandra Burdette Mills

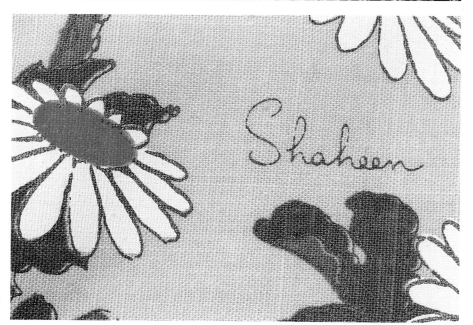

Detail of fabric

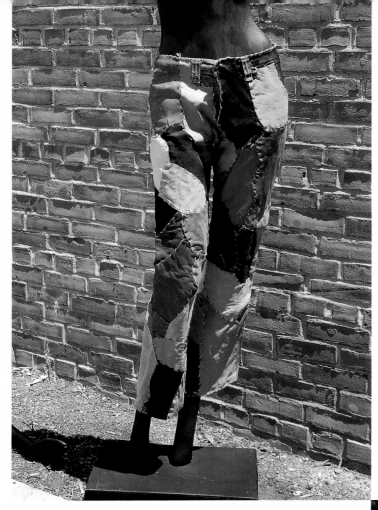

Pant - c. 1960s
Multi-color 100% leather
patches stitched on top of jeans.
$50-$75
Courtesy Shelley Stahlman

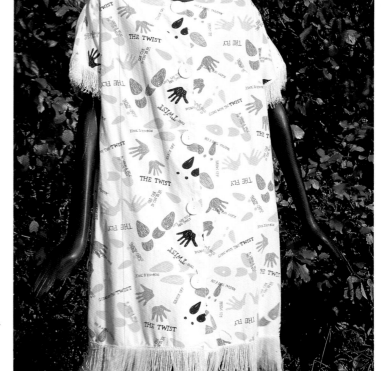

Smock - c. 1960s
White 100% cotton
print with '60s phrases.
$25-$35

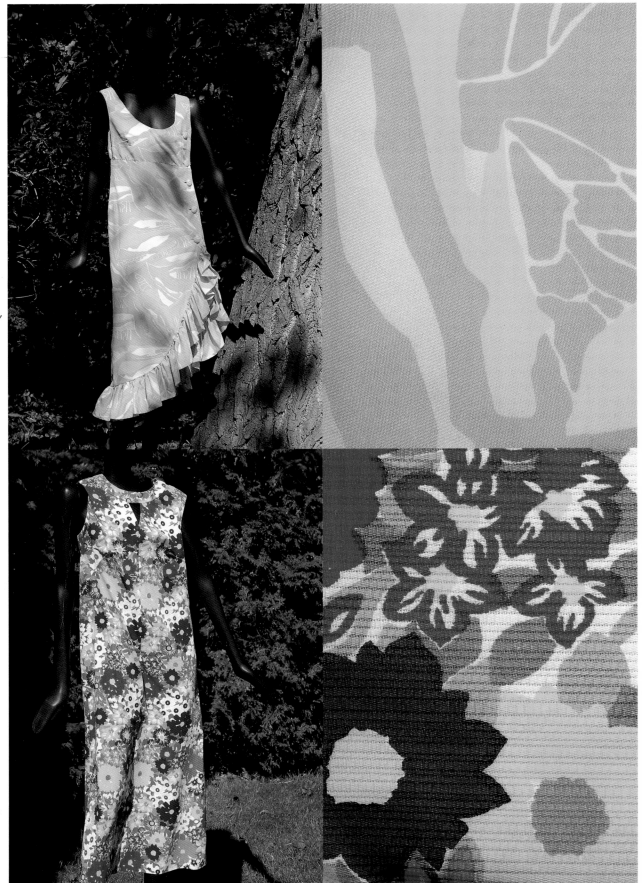

Right:
Hostess dress - c. 1960s
Oriental Fashions, Made in British Hong Kong
Gold print 100% polyester, side button closure, ruffle hem.
$35-$45

Far right:
Detail of fabric

Right:
Hostess dress - c. 1960s
Floral print, 100% cotton, keyhole neckline.
$35-$50

Far right:
Detail of fabric

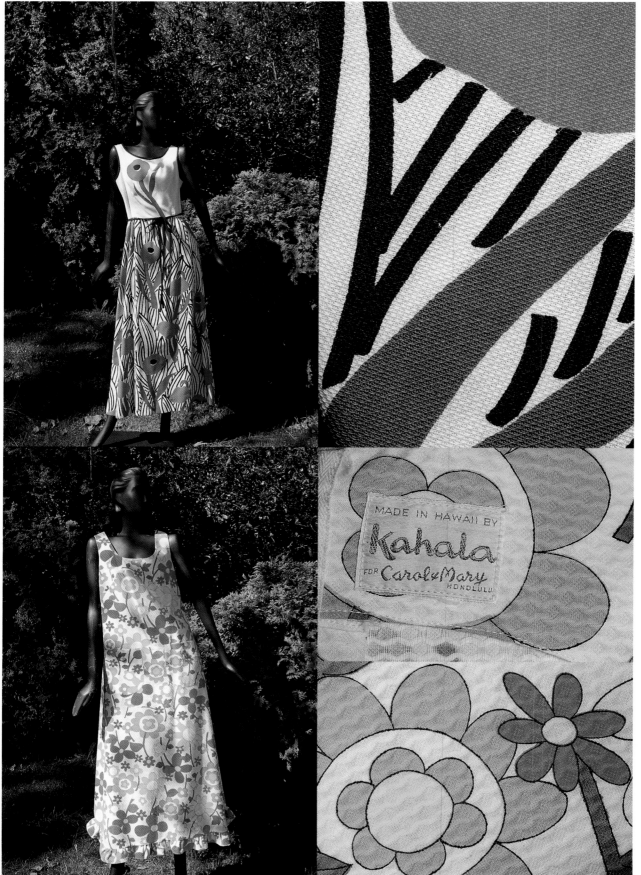

Far left:
Hostess dress - c. 1960s
Tanner of North Carolina
Floral print 100% cotton, poppy motif.
$35-$50

Left:
Detail of fabric

MADE IN HAWAII BY
Kahala
FOR *Carole Mary*
HONOLULU

Left:
Label

Far left:
Hostess dress - c. 1960s
Kahala, Made in Hawaii
Floral print 100% cotton, square neckline, ruffle hem.
$35-$50

Detail of fabric

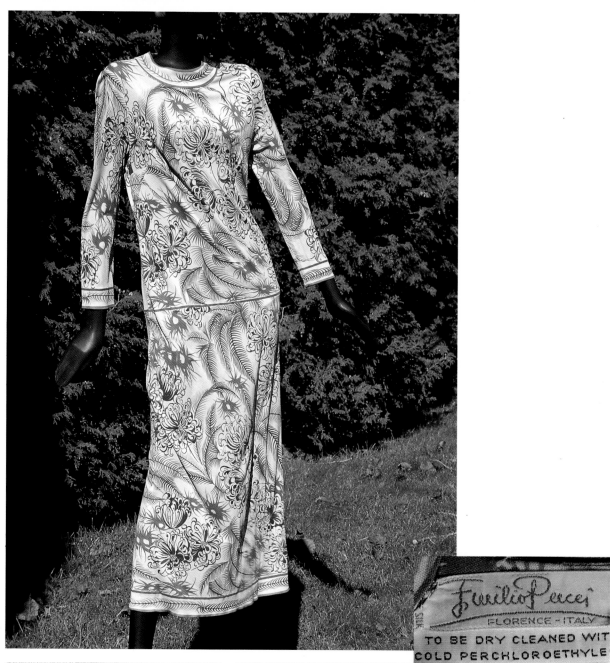

Hostess dress - c.
1960s
Emilio Pucci
Pucci print, 100% silk.
$100-$150

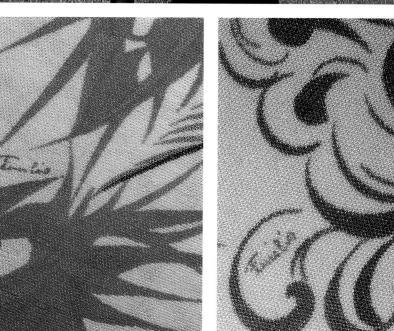

Label

Detail of fabric

Detail of fabric

159

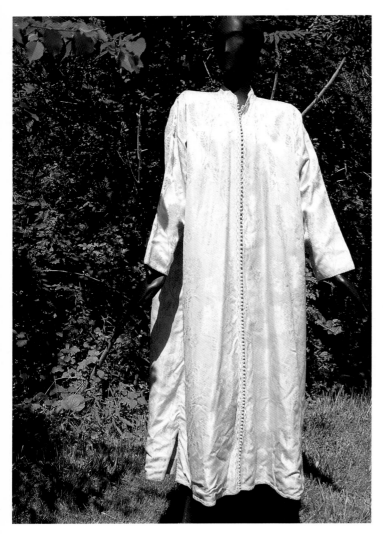

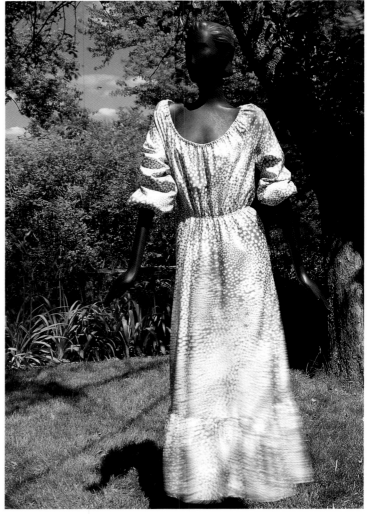

Above:
Caftan - c. 1969
Pale blue 100% silk brocade,
button closure, long sleeve.
$75-$100

Above right:
Hostess dress - c. 1960s
A and O Couture by Artin
Lavender 100% silk print, scoop
neckline, elastic sleeve, ruffle hem.
$40-$60

Right:
Label

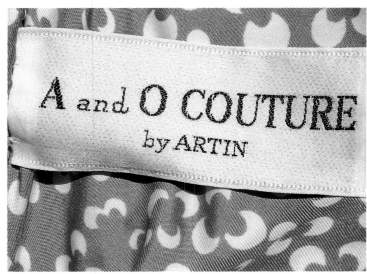

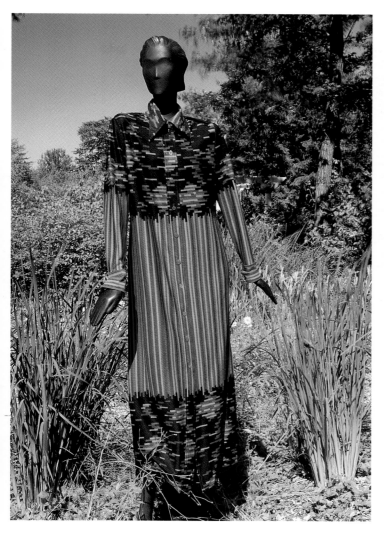

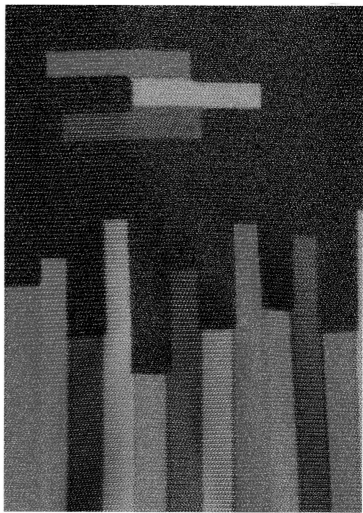

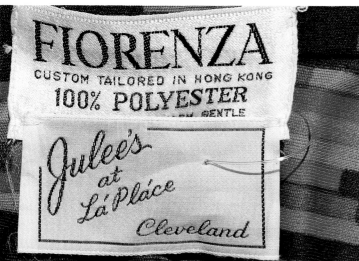

Above left:
Hostess dress - c. 1960s
Fiorenza, Custom Tailored in Hong Kong
Black 100% polyester print, collar,
button closure, long sleeve.
$60-$80

Above right:
Detail of fabric

Left:
Label

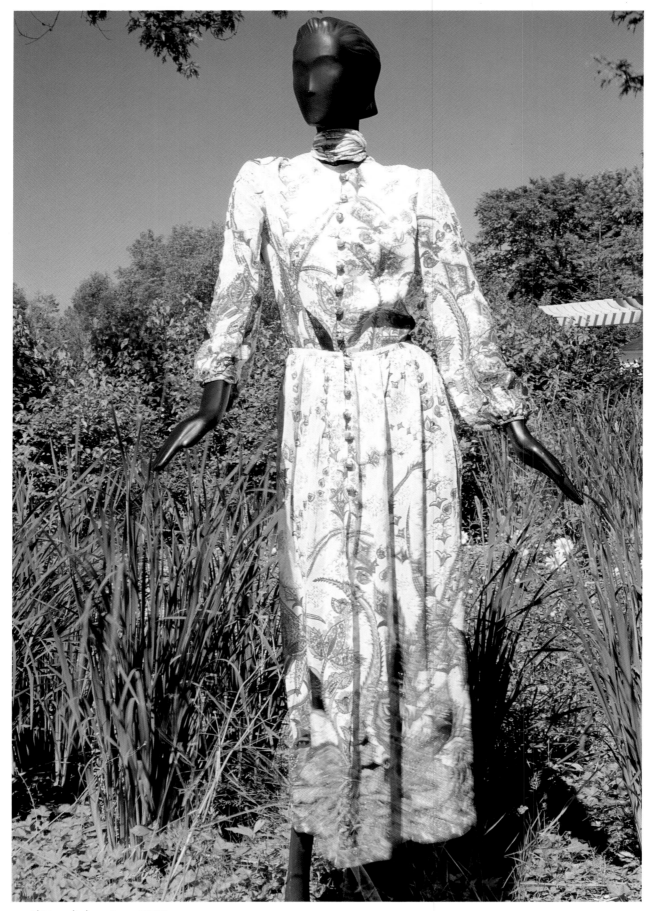

Skirt and playsuit - c. 1960s
Cream 100% silk lamé, bold
print, round neckline, long
skirt, short shorts tunic, shawl.
$75-$100

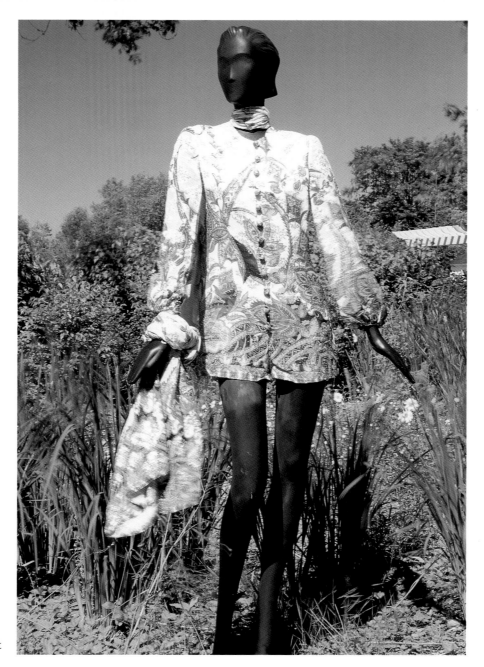

Playsuit

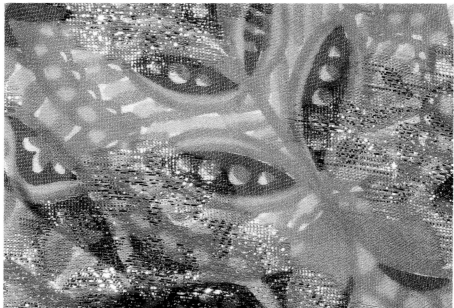

Detail of fabric

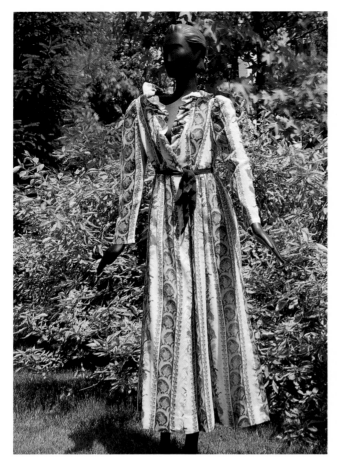

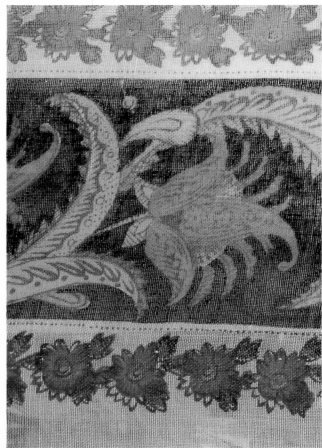

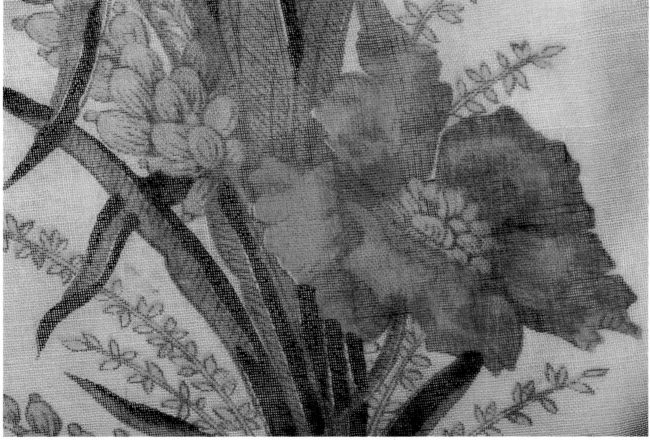

Top left:
Hostess dress - c. 1969
Cream 100% cotton floral print,
ruffle neckline, long sleeve, belted.
$50-$75

Top right and above:
Detail of fabric

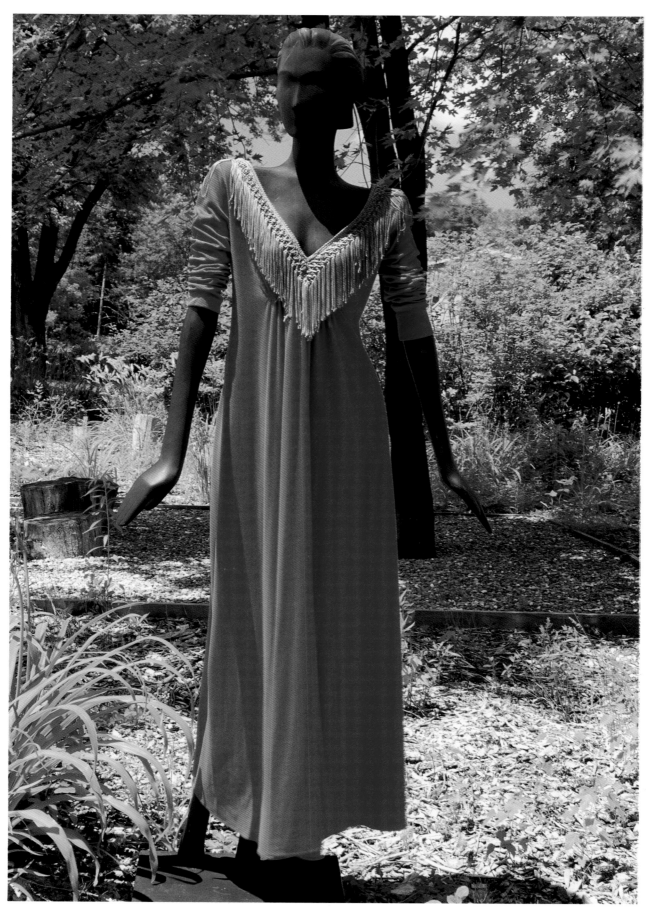

Hostess dress - c. 1968
Red 100% polyester knit, V-neckline,
long sleeve, fringe.
$50-$75

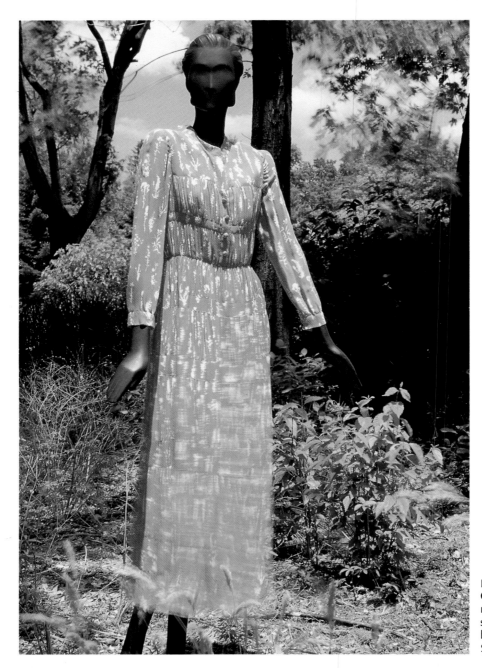

Hostess dress - c. 1968
Coral 100% silk print,
round neckline, bishop
sleeve, button closure,
banded gathered skirt.
$50-$75

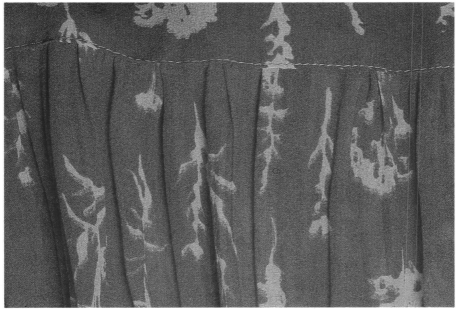

Detail of fabric

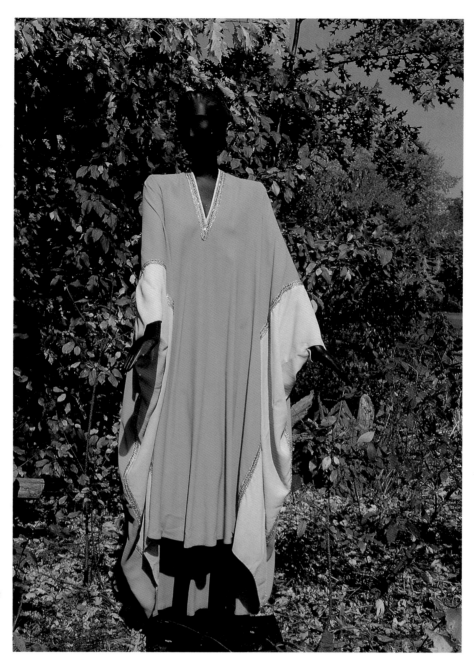

Caftan - c. 1960s
Jay Morley for Fern Violette
Green and pink 100%
polyester, gold braid trim.
$60-$80
Courtesy Studio Moderne

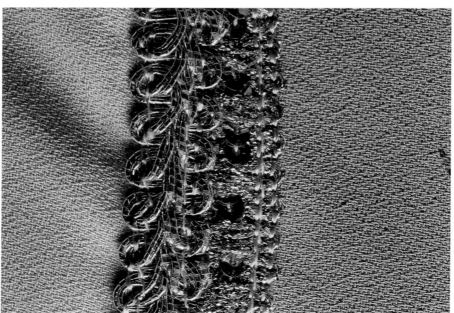

Detail of fabric

167

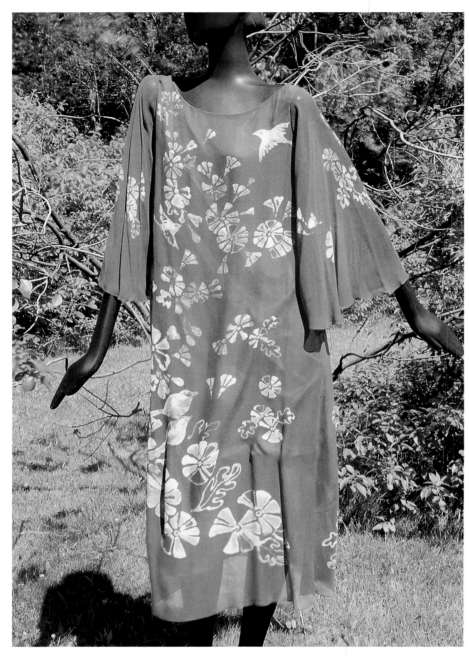

Hostess dress - c. 1968
Brown 100% silk, hand
painted flower, scoop
neckline, trumpet sleeve.
$100-$150

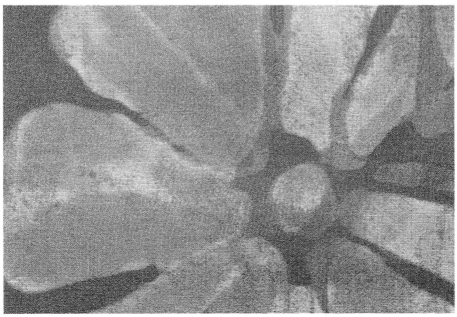

Detail of fabric

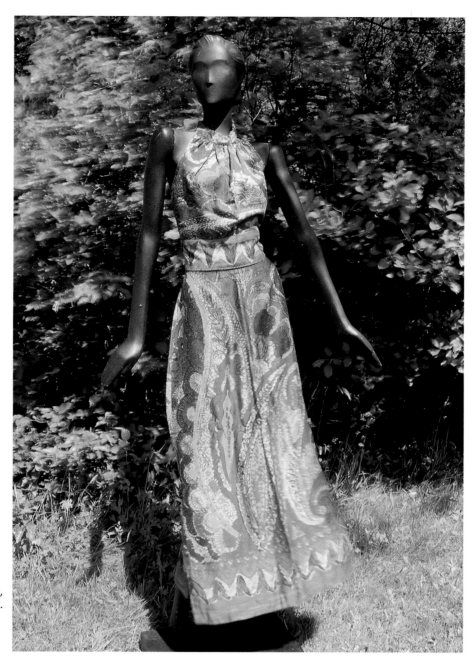

Top and skirt - c. 1960s
Turquoise 100% cotton
multi bold print, halter top,
gathered waistline, side slit.
$50-$75
*Courtesy Sandra Burdette
Mills*

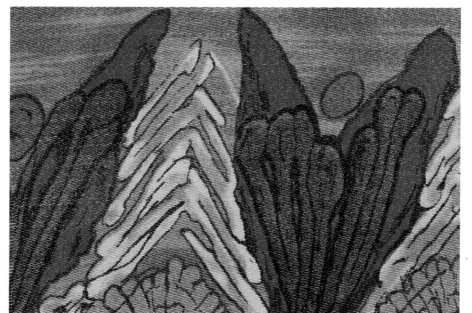

Detail of fabric

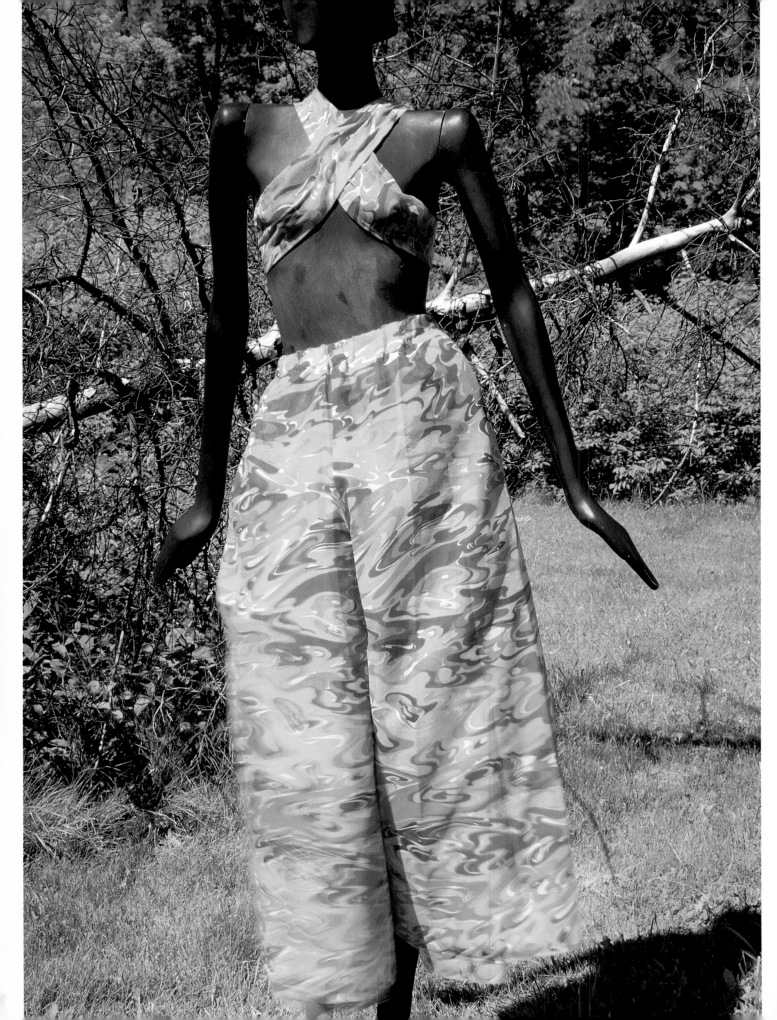

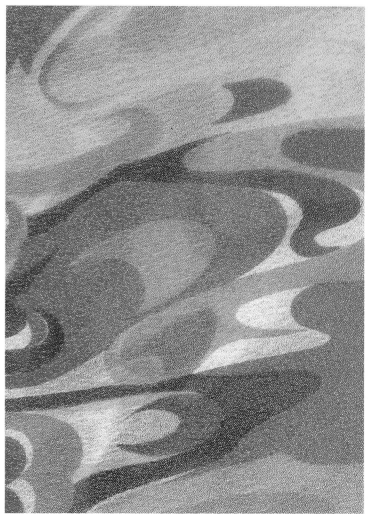

Detail of fabric

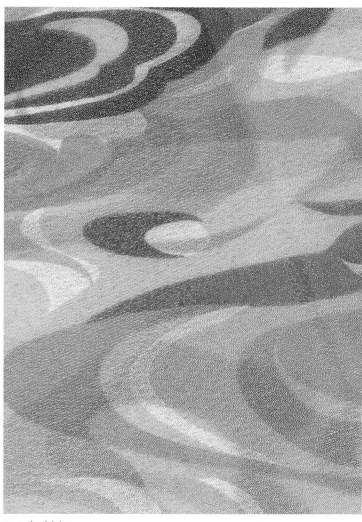

Detail of fabric

Opposite:
Pant - c. 1960s
Orange 100% silk, oil slick motif,
side leg slit, elastic waistline.
$50-$75
Courtesy Sandra Burdette Mills

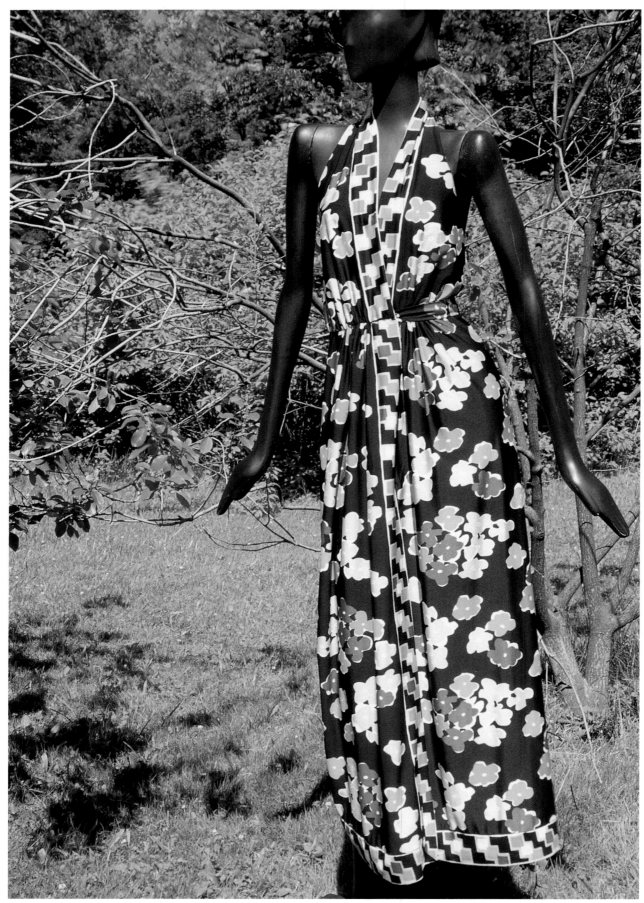

Hostess dress - c. 1960s
Oscar de la Renta
Navy 100% polyester print,
halter bodice, tie closure.
$100-$150

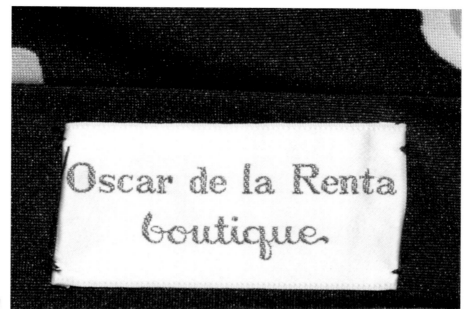

Label

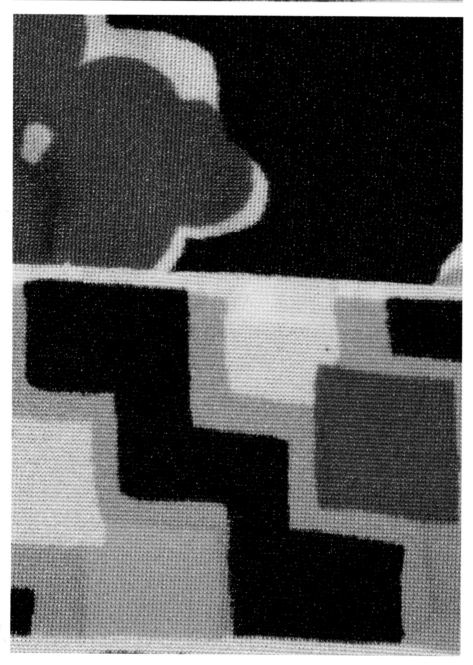

Detail of fabric

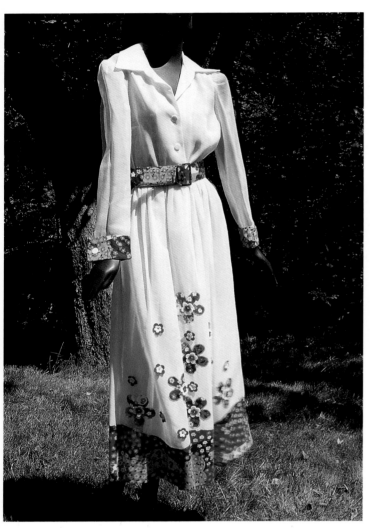

Hostess dress - c. 1960s
White 100% cotton print
appliqué, notched collar,
belted shirtwaist, border hem.
$50-$75

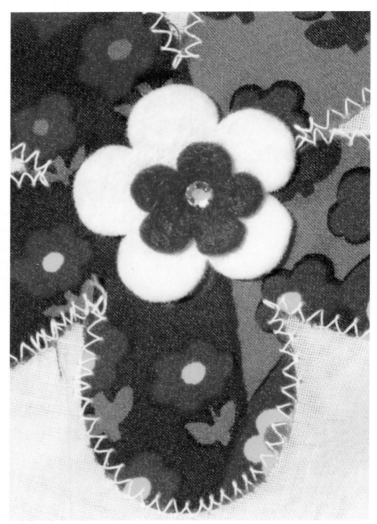

Detail of appliqué

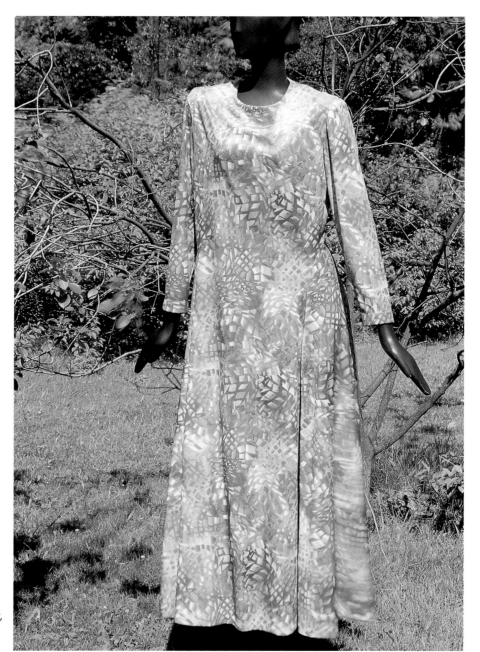

Hostess dress - c. 1969
Umba for Parues
Feinstein, Julee's at Lá
Pláce, Cleveland
Green 100% polyester
multi-print, round collar,
long sleeve.
$50-$75

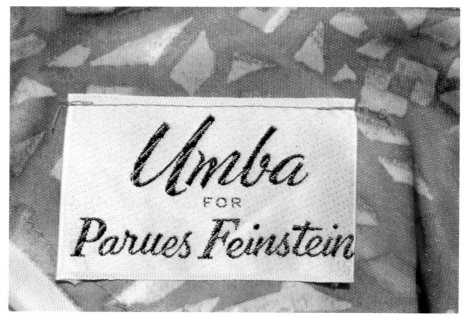

Label

175

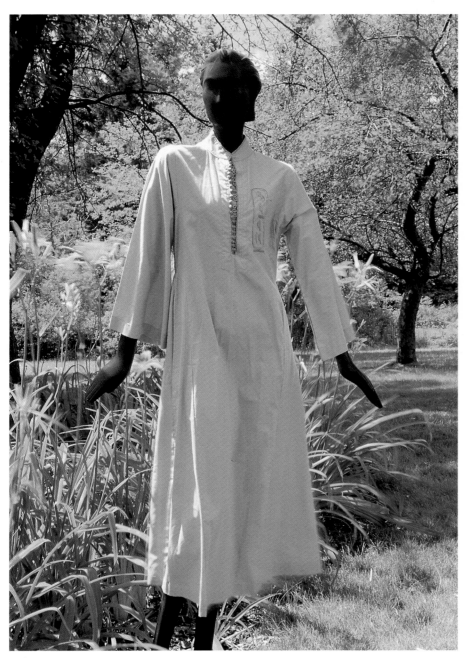

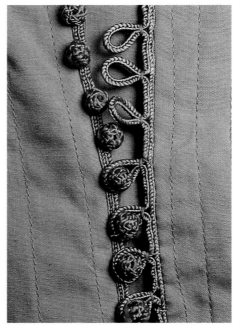

Detail of button

Caftan - c. 1969
Blue lavender 100% cotton,
mandarin collar, crochet
button closure.
$50-$75

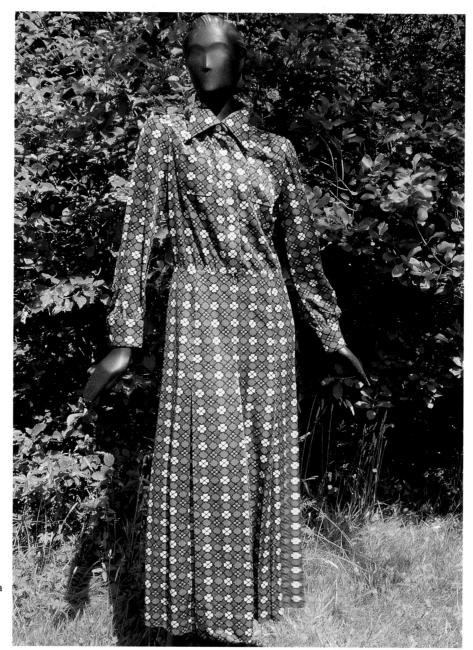

Hostess dress - c. 1960s
Suzy Perette by Victor Costa
Multi 100% silk, geometric
print collar, long sleeve,
button closure.
$100-$150

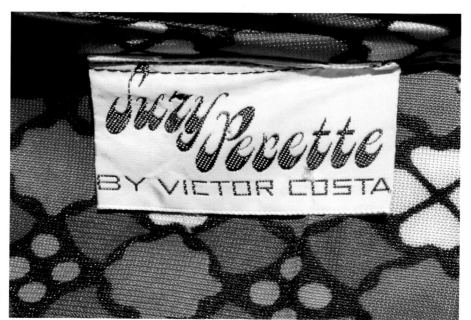

Label

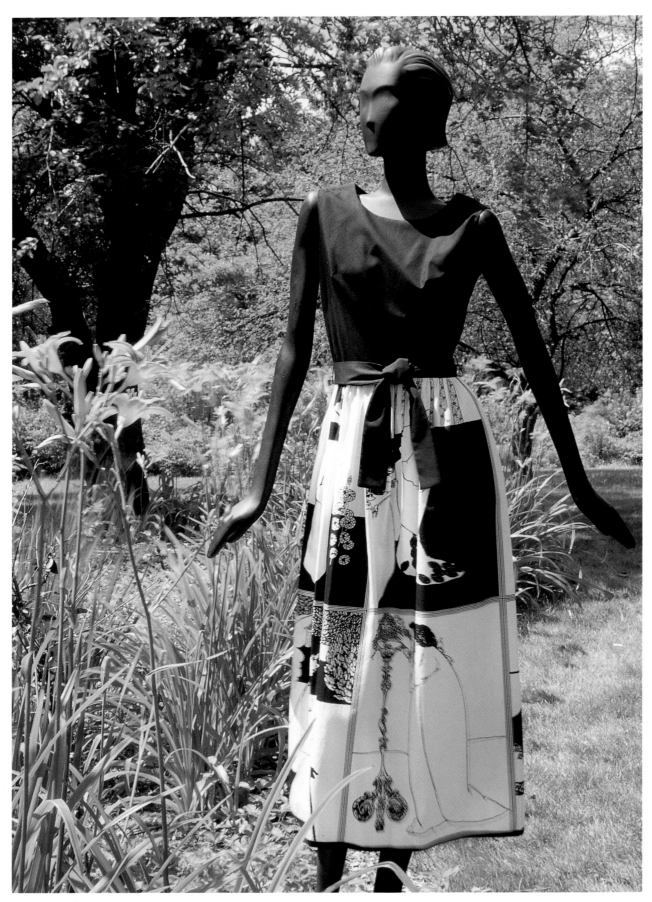

Hostess dress - c. 1960s
Joan Curtin Original
Black and white 100% cotton Aubrey Beardsley Art Nouveau
revival print, scoop neckline, sleeveless.
$100-$150
Courtesy Shirley Friedland

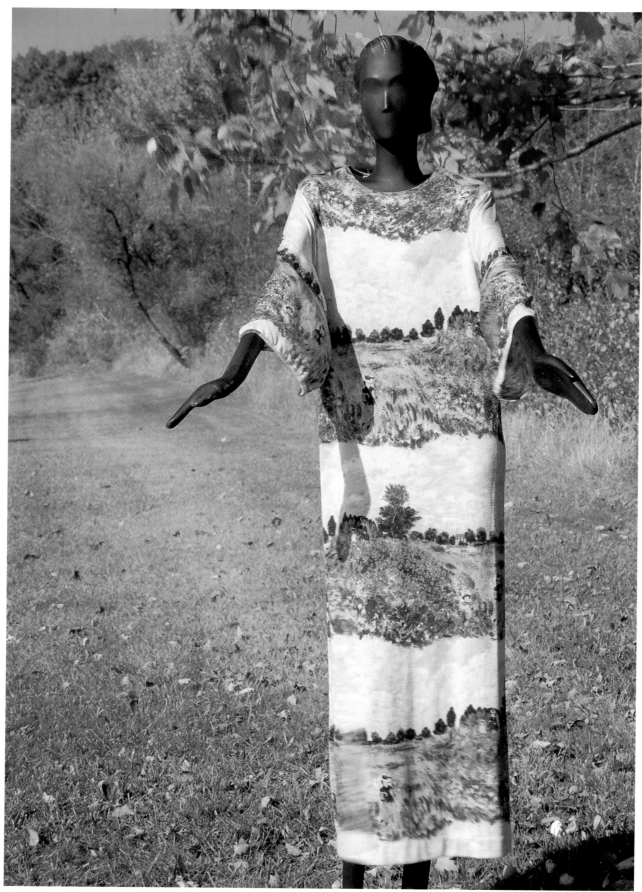

Hostess dress - c. 1960s
Goldworm, Italy
Claude Monet Impressionist print 100% cotton knit.
$100-$150

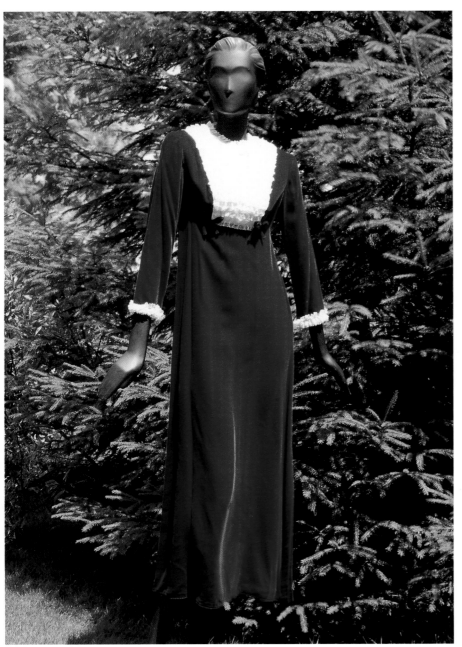

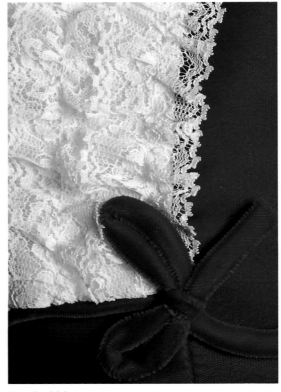

Detail of fabric

Hostess Dress - c. 1960s
Maroon 100% velvet, round neckline,
lace bodice, empire waistline, slim skirt.
$75-$95

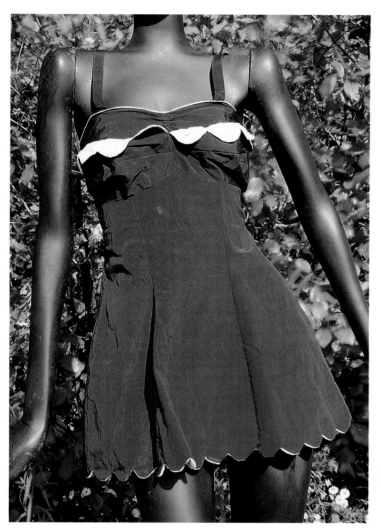

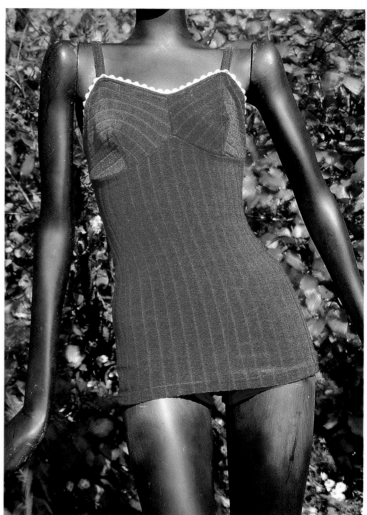

Swimsuit - c. 1950s
Catalina, Styled for the Stars of Hollywood
Navy 100% Spandex, scallop bodice and skirt.
$25-$35

Swimsuit - c. 1950s
Red 100% polyester knit, white trim
bodice and front modesty panel..
$25-$35

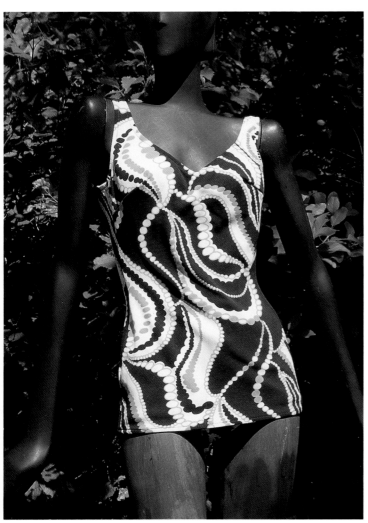

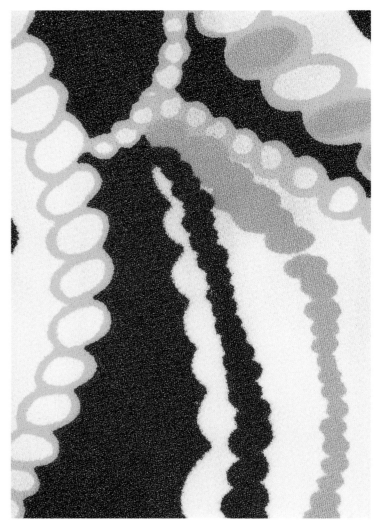

Swimsuit - c. 1960s
Robby Len Fashions
Brown, white and orange 100% stretch nylon,
bold print with snap in bodice (You're a"SNAP"
away from a better silhouette when you buy your
snap in "Shape-lee") and front modesty panel.
$25-$35

Detail of fabric

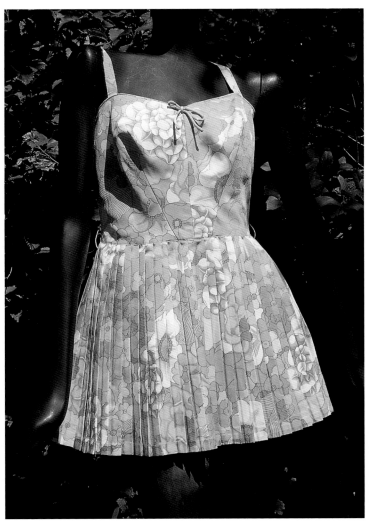

Swimsuit - c. 1960s
GaBar, New York
Pink 100% nylon, floral print, fitted
bodice with stretch side panel,
pleated skirt and pink bloomer.
$25-$35

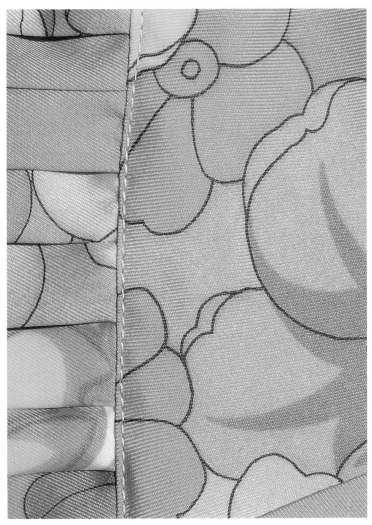

Detail of fabric

Chapter 6

Evening

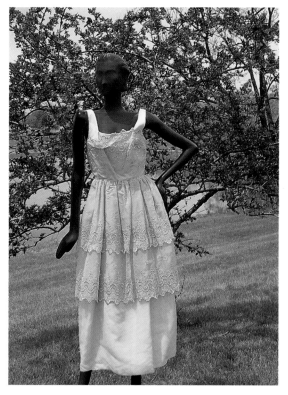

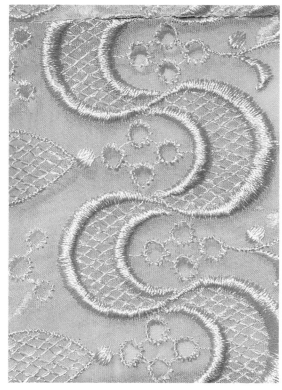

Far left:
Evening dress - c. 1950s
Blue 100% silk, embroidery overlay bodice, square neckline, layered flounce skirt.
$75-$100

Left:
Detail of fabric

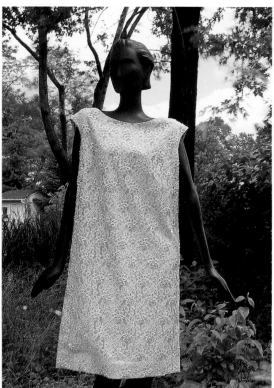

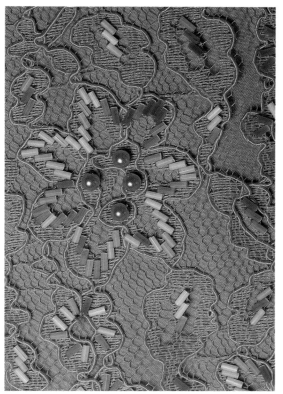

Far left:
Evening dress - c. 1950s
Andora, Hand Fashioned in Hong Kong
Blue 100% rayon, scoop neckline, cap sleeve, beaded net overlay.
$70-$90

Left:
Detail of fabric

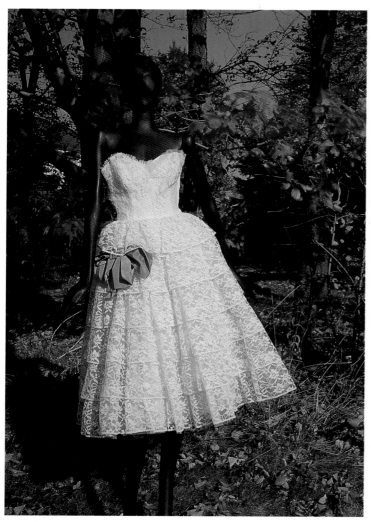

Evening dress - c. 1950s
Peach 100% nylon net, rumba ruffle
formal, boned bodice, bow at hip.
$50-$75

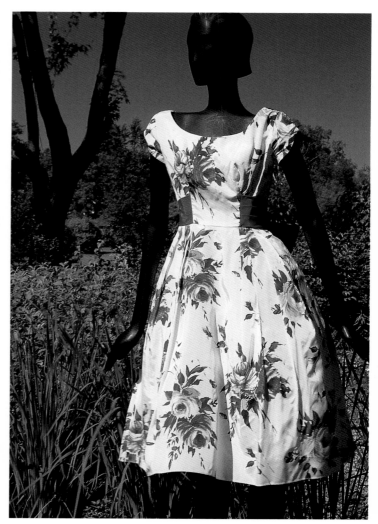

Evening dress - c. 1959
Floral 100% rayon, rose print,
scoop neckline, cap sleeve,
bodice sash, pleated skirt.
$40-$60

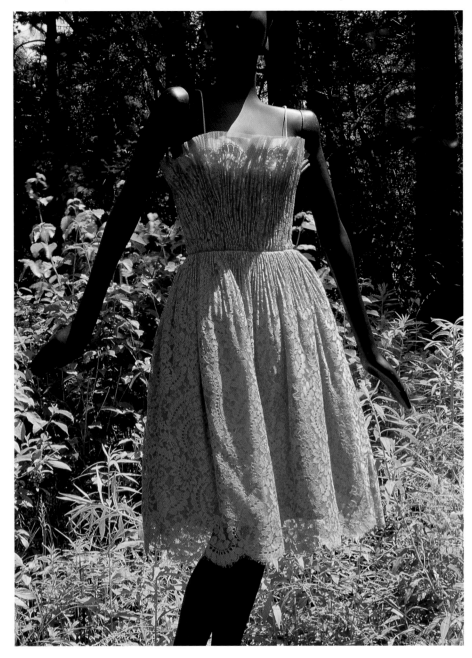

Evening dress - c. 1950s
Rose lace pleated bodice, gathered skirt.
$75-$100

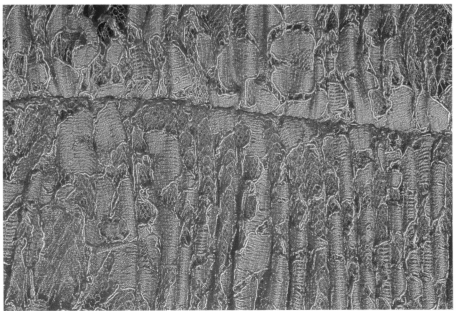

Detail of fabric

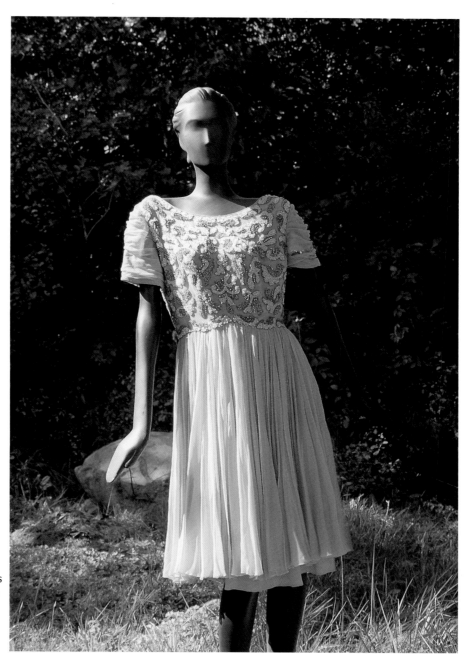

Evening dress - c. 1950s
Gold 100% silk chiffon,
beaded bodice, scoop
neckline, cap sleeve,
gathered skirt.
$150-$175

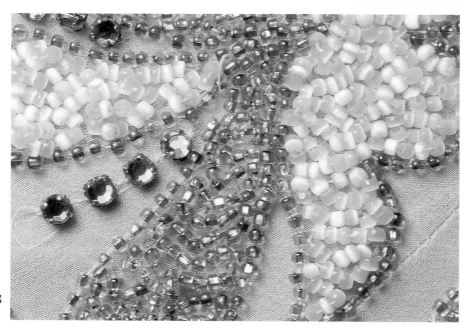

Detail of beading

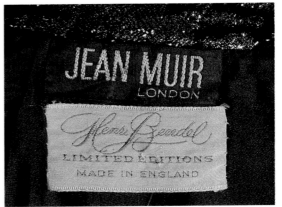

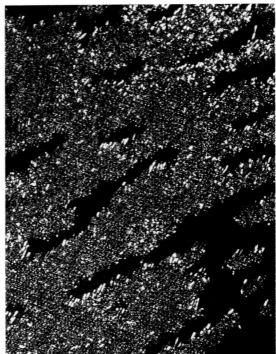

Detail of fabric

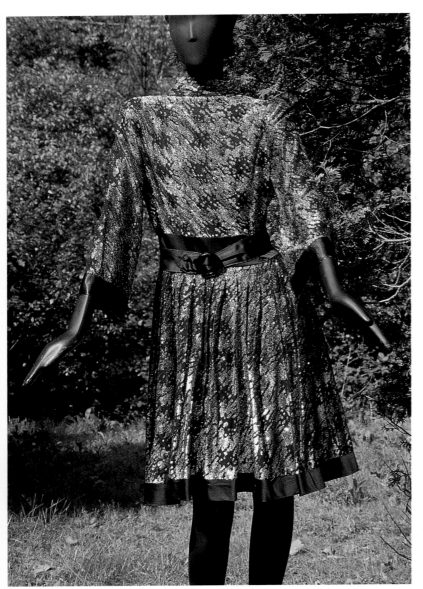

Evening dress - c. 1958
Jean Muir, London; Henri Bendel
Limited Editions, Made in England
Silver 100% voided lamé, standing
collar, long sleeve, black satin
waistline, gathered skirt.
$100-$125

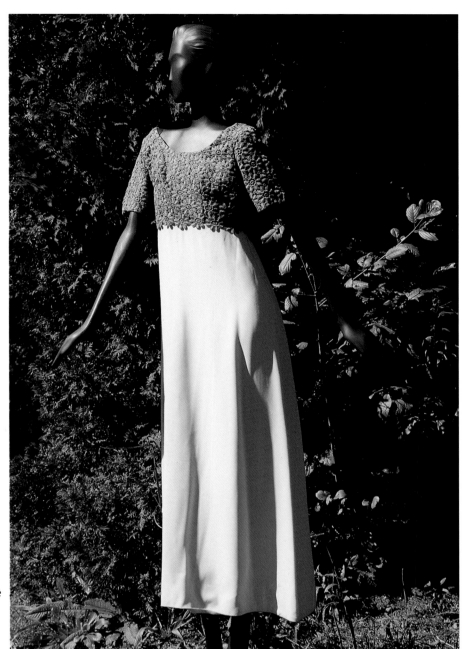

Evening dress - c. 1950s
Cream 100% silk, olive lace
bodice, cap sleeve, empire
waistline, slim skirt, panel
back.
$75-$100

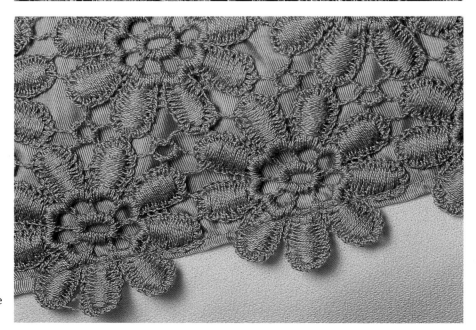

Detail of lace

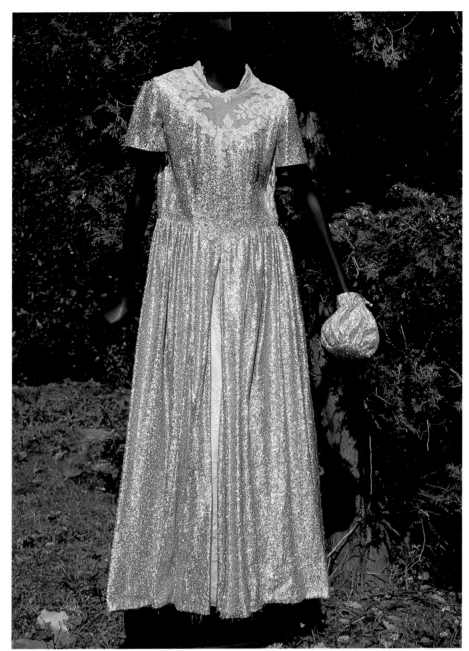

Evening gown - c. 1950s
Ann's Vogue Shoppe,
Cleveland, Ohio
Gold silk lamé, lace
appliqué bodice, short
sleeve, gathered full skirt
with matching draw string
handbag.
$100-$150

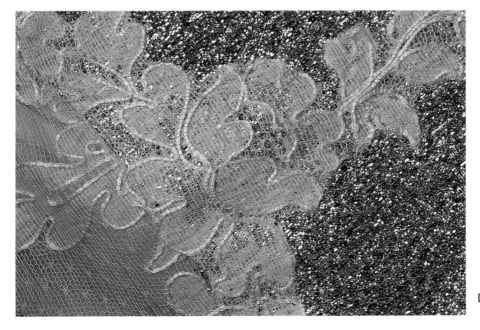

Detail of fabric

190

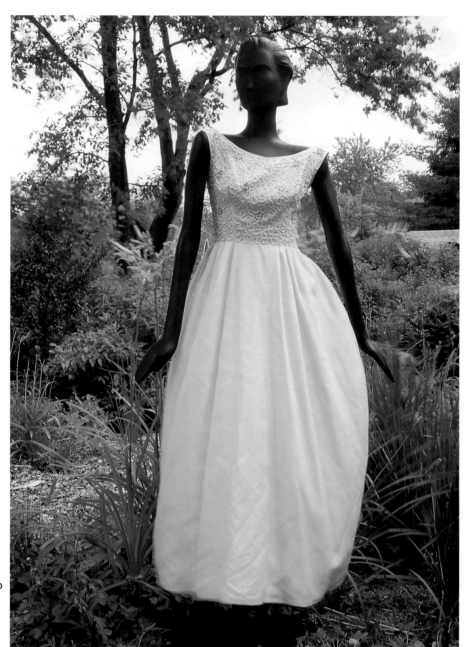

Evening gown - c. 1950s
Yellow 100% nylon, scoop
neckline, sleeveless,
braided bodice, pleated
long skirt.
$50-$75

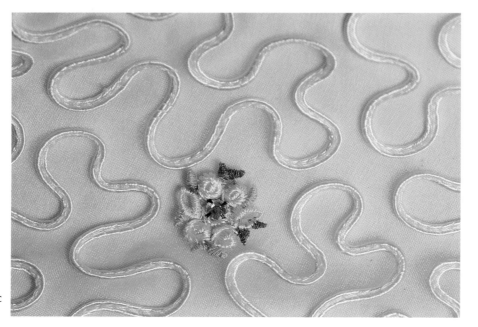

Detail of fabric

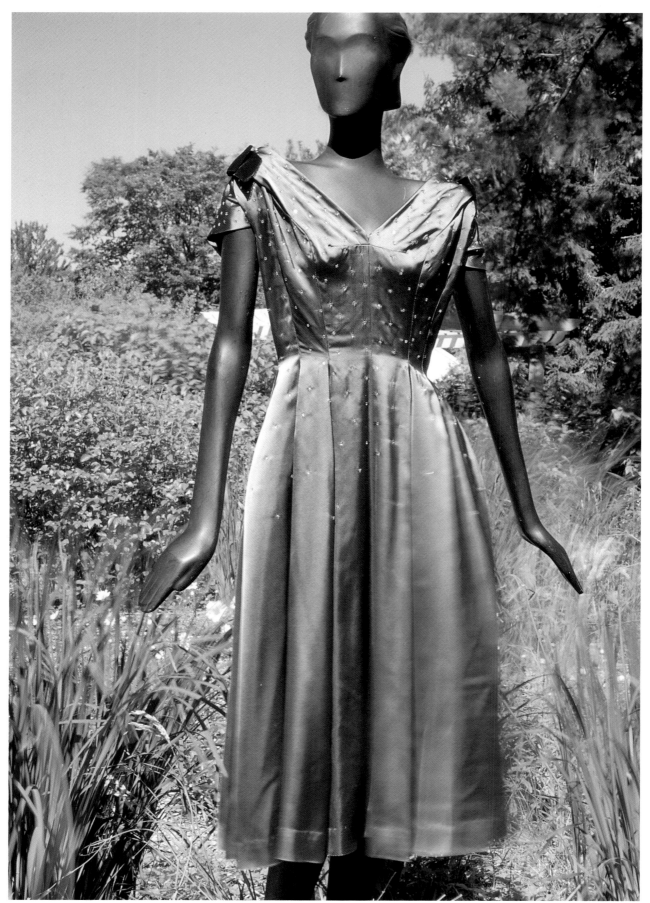

Evening dress - c. 1950s
Purple 100% silk satin, V-neckline, cap sleeve, rhinestone bodice, velvet shoulder bow, full circle skirt.
$100-$150

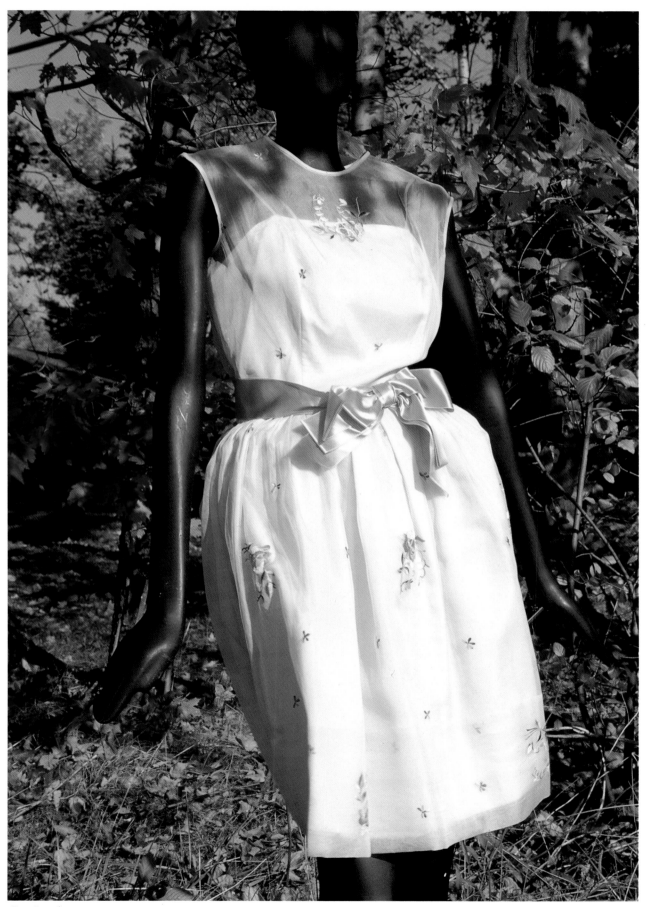

Evening dress - c. 1950s
Cream 100% silk organza, sheer bodice,
embroidery, gathered skirt, pink satin bow belt.
$60-$80

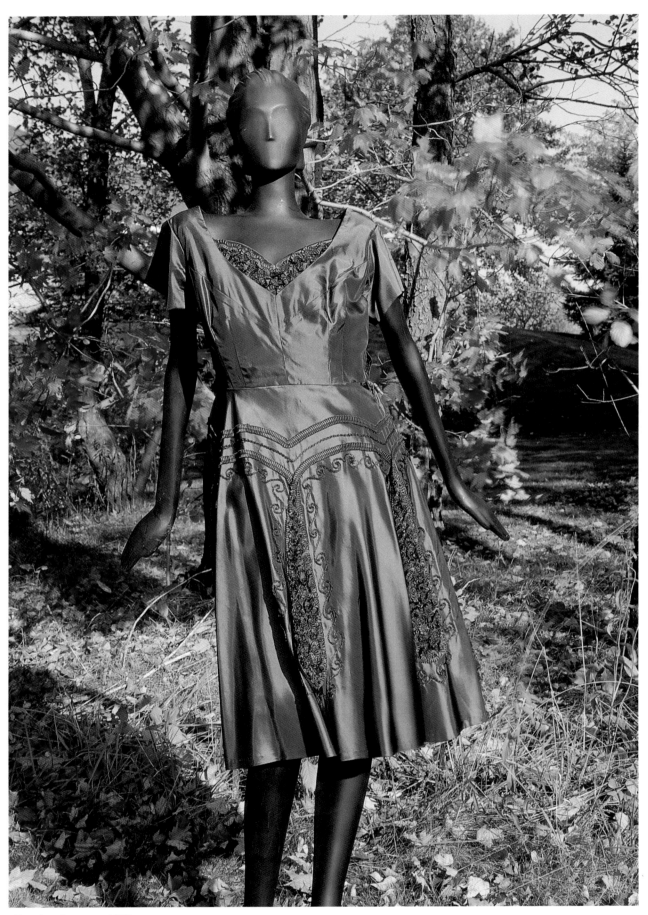

Evening dress - c. 1950s
Lisieux Shop, Pittsfield, MA
Purple 100% rayon, sweetheart neckline,
cap sleeve, ribbon trim, full skirt.
$50-$75

Evening dress - c. 1950s
Harry Keiser
Red velvet, sweetheart neckline,
gathered sleeve, full circle skirt.
$60-$80

Evening dress - c. 1950s
London's, Erie
Green satin, round collar, 3/4 sleeve,
rhinestone button closure, pleated skirt.
$60-$80

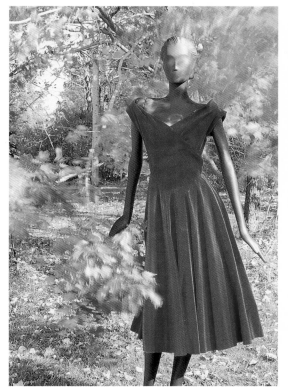

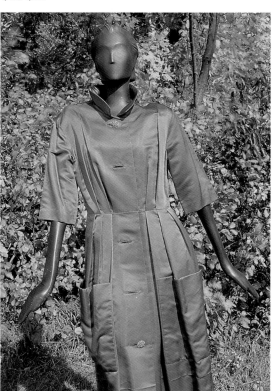

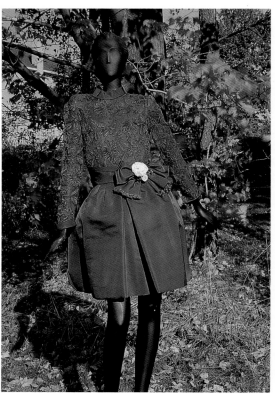

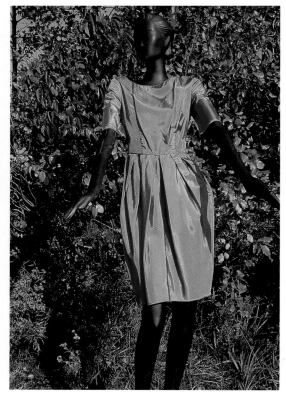

Evening dress - c. 1950s
Chester Weinberg, Edward Hurwitch, Hartford
Olive 100% silk, lace bodice, bouffant skirt, sash
rose tie.
$100-$150

Evening dress - c. 1950s
Orange 100% rayon, scoop
neckline, 3/4 sleeve, pleated skirt.
$40-$60

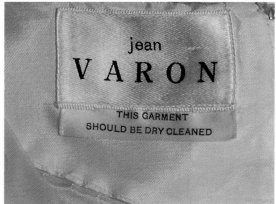

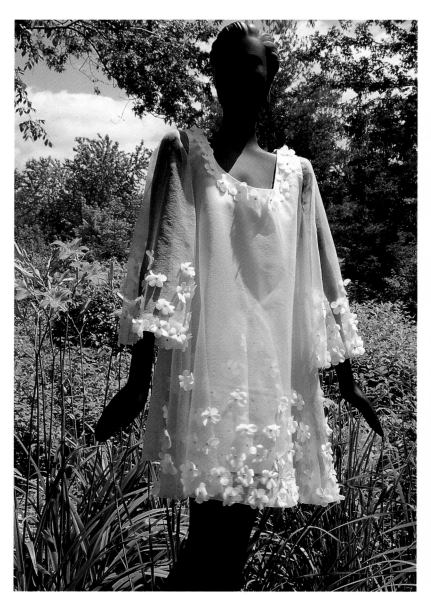

Evening dress - c. 1960s
Jean Varon, Made in England
Pink 100% nylon, scoop neckline,
trumpet sleeve, white flower appliqué,
A-line silhouette.
$70-$90

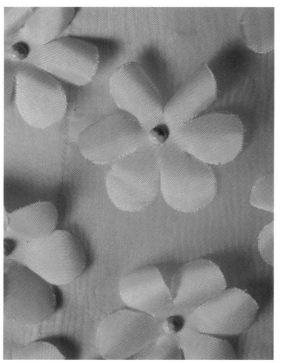

Detail of flower appliqué

Opposite:

Top left: Evening dress - c. 1960s
Cathay Imports Limited
White 100% silk, scoop neckline, sleeveless,
rhinestone trim, mini silhouette.
$60-$80

Top right: Detail of rhinestone

Bottom left: Evening dress - c. 1960s
Beige 100% lace, scoop neckline, cap sleeve,
pearl rhinestone sequin overlay.
$100-$150

Bottom right: Detail of fabric

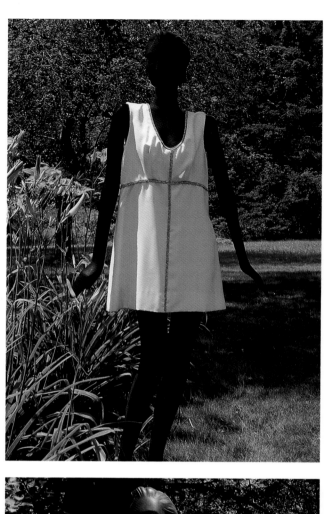

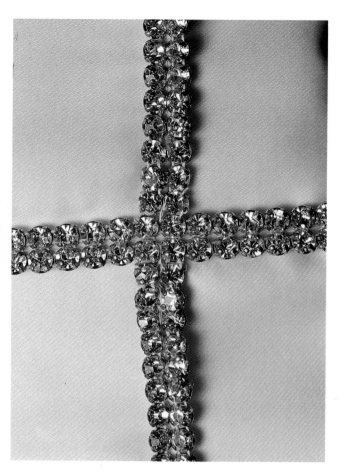

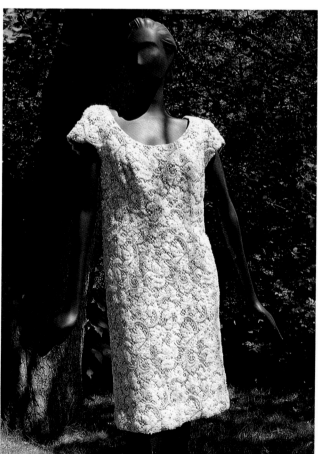

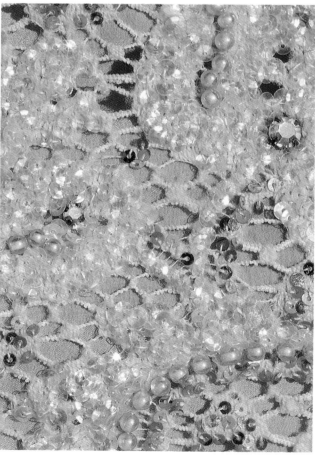

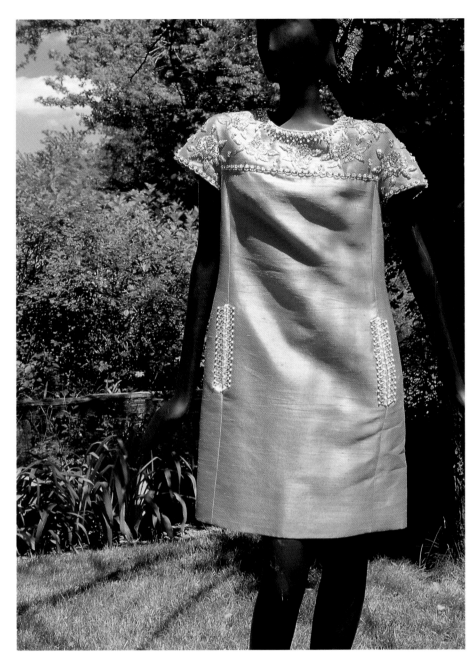

Evening dress - c. 1960s
Hot pink 100% silk, round
neckline, short sleeve,
pearl rhinestone beaded
yoke and pocket.
$100-$150

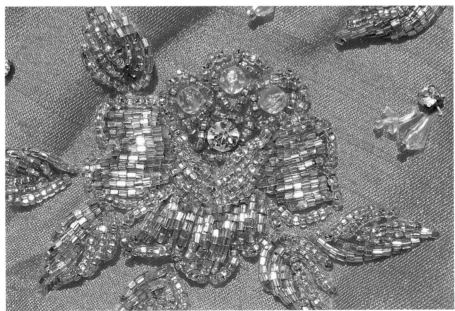

Detail of beading

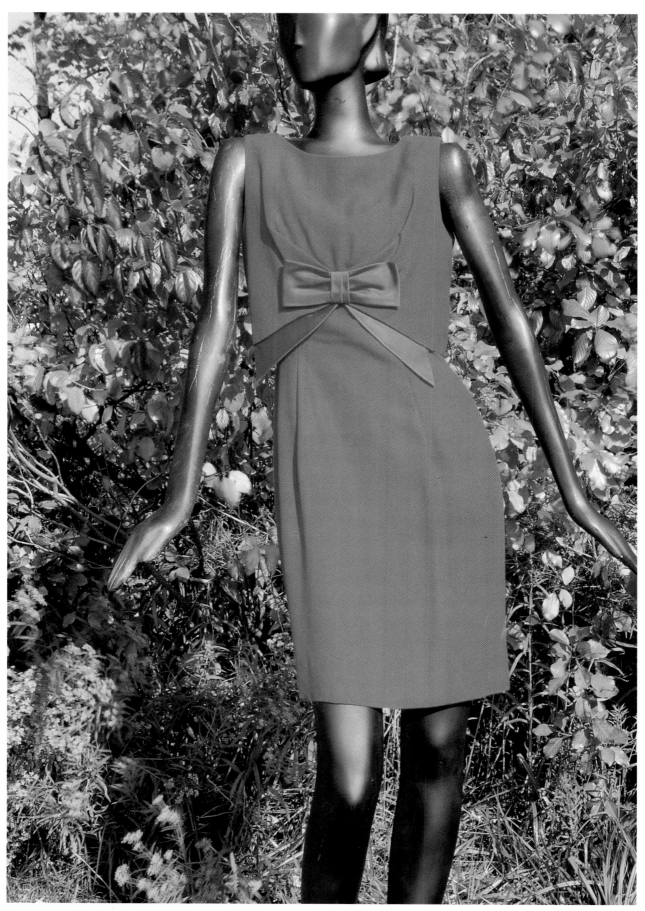

Evening dress - c. 1960s
Raspberry 100% silk, scoop neckline,
sleeveless, bow bodice, straight skirt.
$50-$75

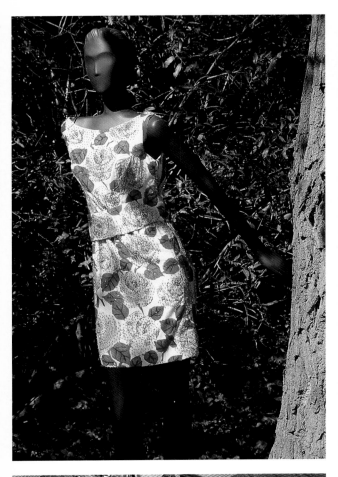

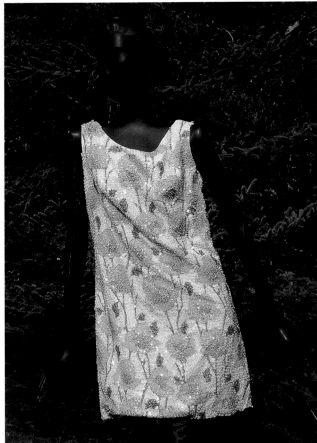

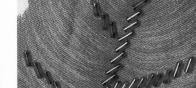

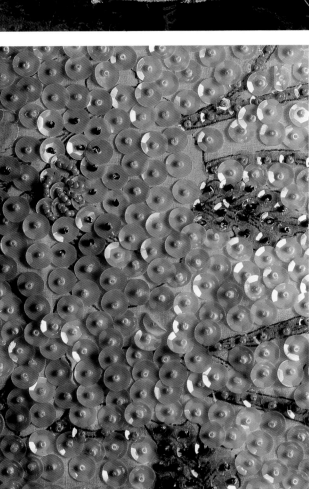

Detail of fabric

Detail of fabric

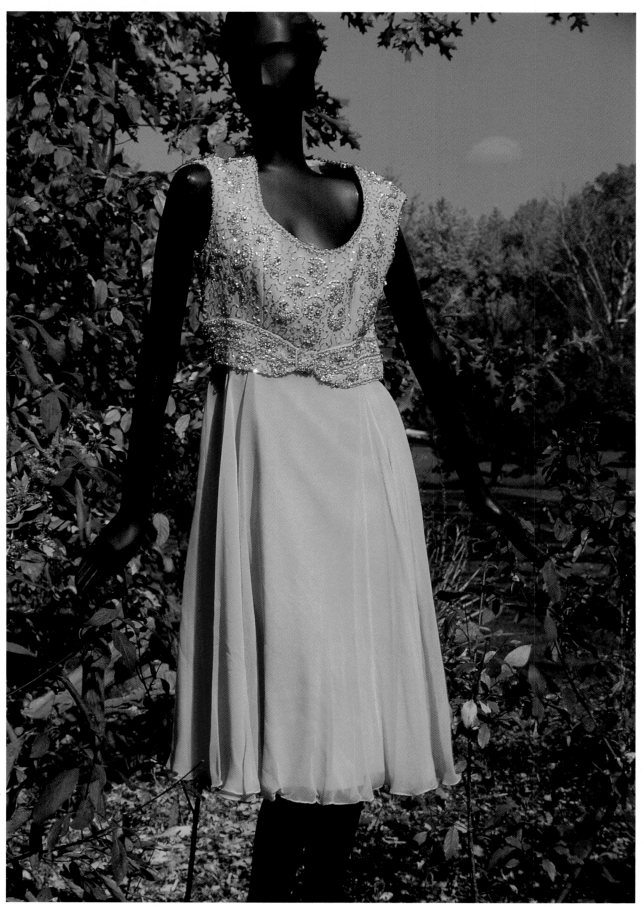

Evening dress - c. 1960s
Orange 100% silk chiffon, scoop neckline,
sleeveless, beaded bodice, gathered skirt.
$100-$150
Courtesy Studio Moderne

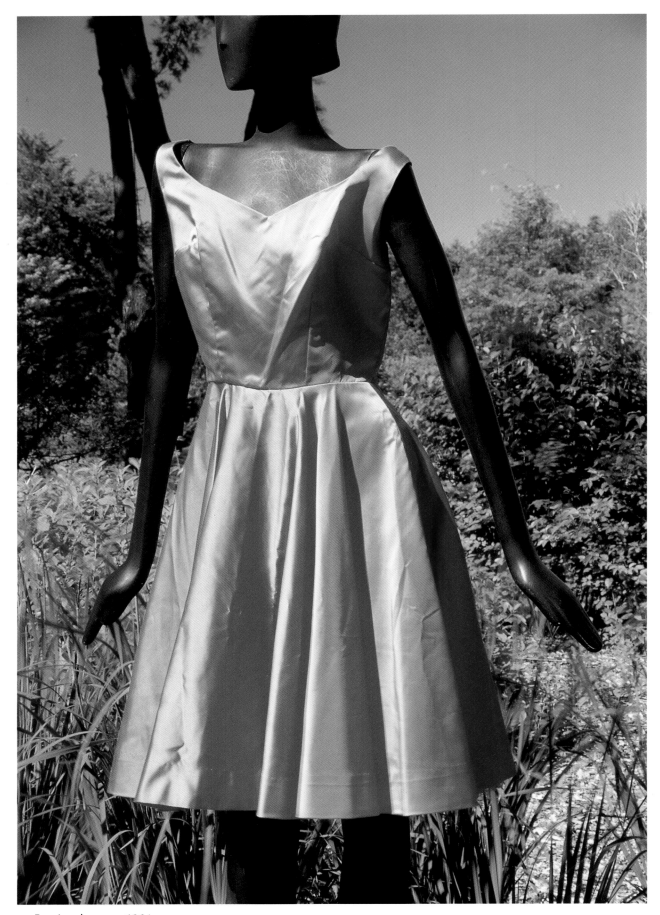

Evening dress - c. 1964
Coral 100% silk satin, scoop
neckline, sleeveless, full circle skirt.
$50-$75
Courtesy Barbara Johnson Cook

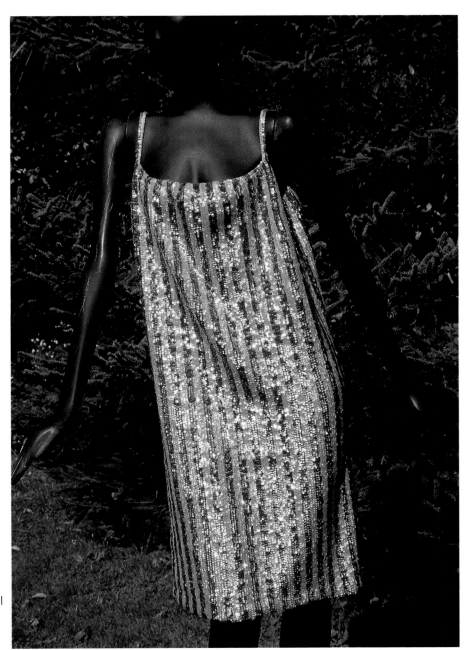

Evening dress - c. 1960s
Pink and green knit,
covered with sequins,
straight neckline, straps, full
silhouette.
$100-$125
Courtesy Studio Moderne

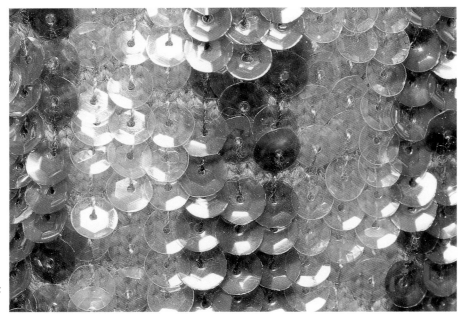

Detail of fabric

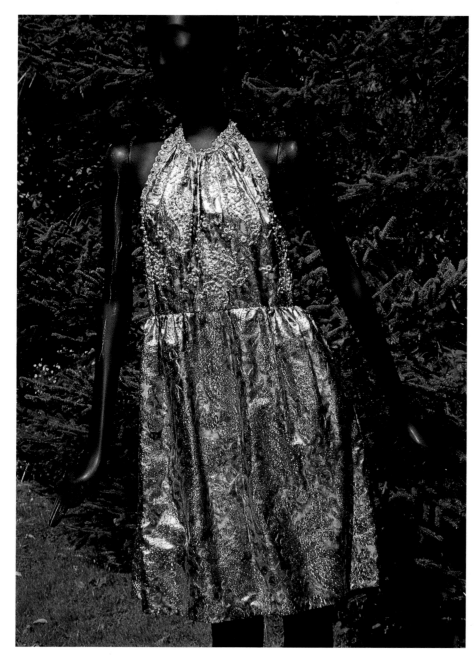

Evening dress - c. 1960s
Morton Myles for Malcolm
Charles
Gold, green and blue metallic
silk halter bodice, braid at
neckline, gathered skirt.
$100-$150
Courtesy Studio Moderne

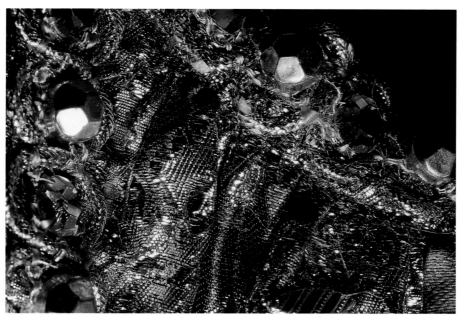

Detail of fabric

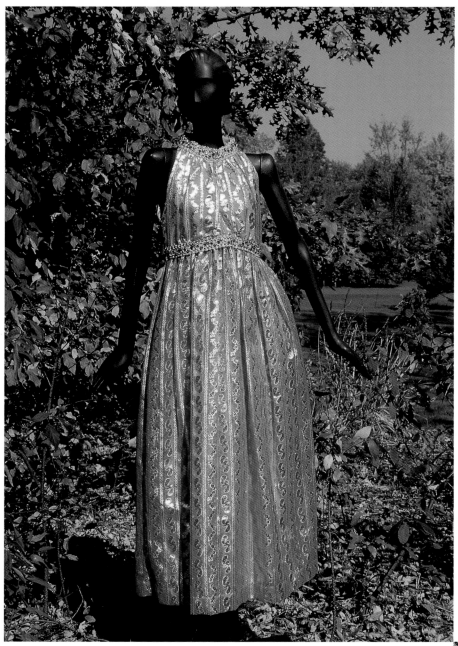

Above:
Evening dress - c. 1960s
Morton Myles for Malcolm
Charles, Higbee Co.
Orange and metallic gold
paisley halter bodice, braid
at waistline, gathered skirt.
$100-$150
Courtesy Studio Moderne

Right:
Detail of fabric

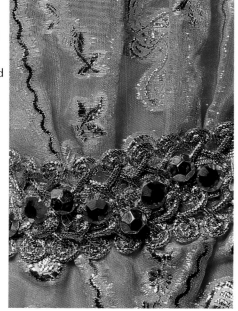

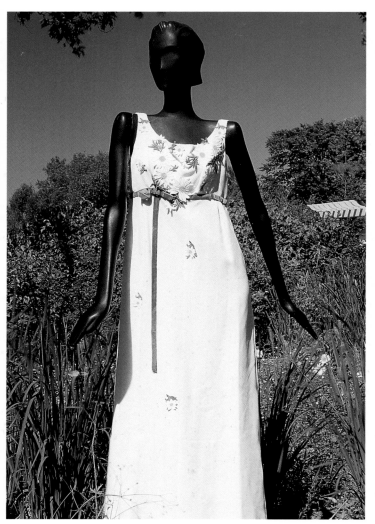

Evening dress - c. 1960s
White 100% silk, scoop neckline,
sleeveless, empire waistline, daisy
appliqué, straight skirt.
$50-$75

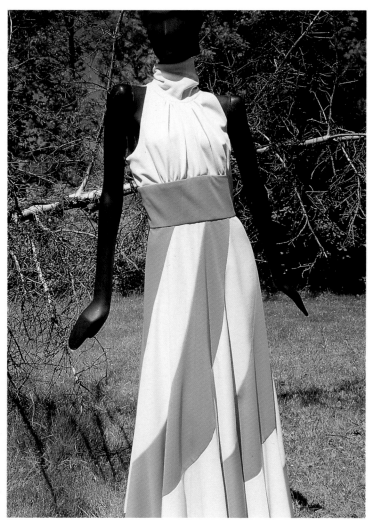

Evening dress - c. 1960s
Cream and green 100% polyester
knit, halter neckline, sleeveless,
cummerbund waistline, diagonal
bias drape skirt scallop hem.
$100-$150
Courtesy Elaine Doman Johnson

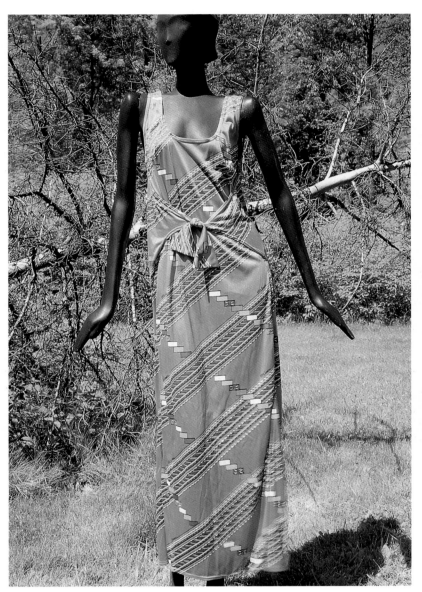

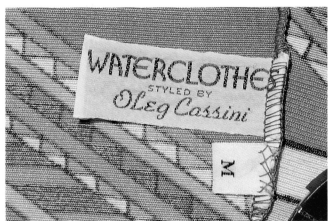

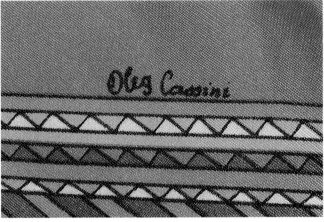

Evening dress - c. 1960s
Waterclothes Styled by Oleg Cassini
Green 100% polyester knit, geometric
print, scoop neckline, sleeveless,
bodice front wrap, pencil skirt.
$100-$150
Courtesy Elaine Doman Johnson

Top:
Label

Above:
Detail of fabric

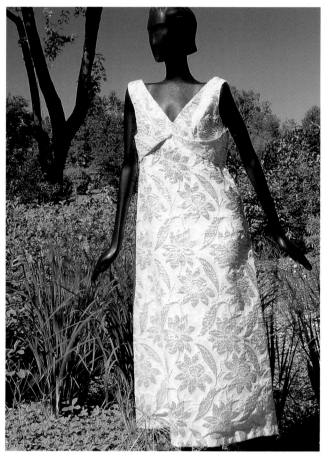

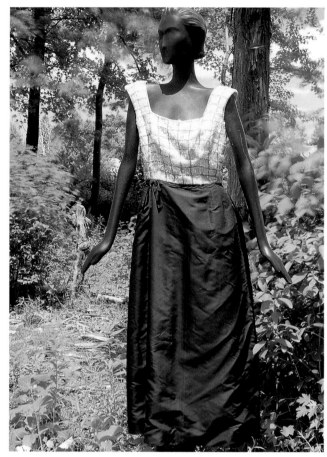

Above:
Evening dress - c. 1969
Silver lamé, V-neckline,
sleeveless, empire waistline
and A-line silhouette.
$50-$75

Above right:
Evening gown - c. 1960s
Long black satin skirt, square
neckline, sleeveless, sequin
bodice.
$75-$125

Right:
Detail of fabric

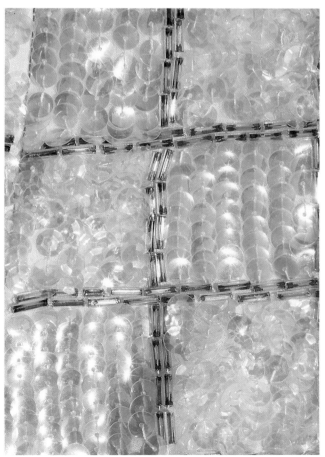

Evening gown - c. 1970
Silver 100% silk, round neckline, sleeveless,
rhinestone pearl crystal beaded yoke, empire
waistline, slim skirt.
$150-$175

Detail of yoke

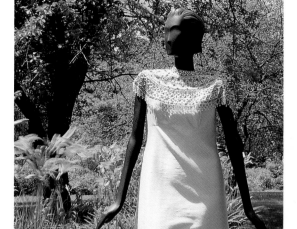

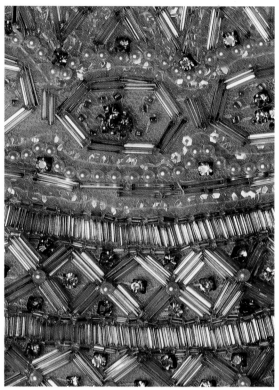

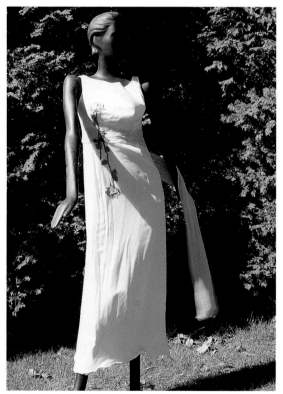

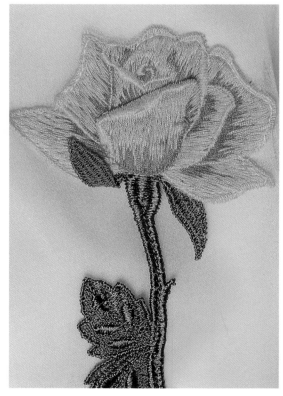

Evening dress - c. 1960s
White 100% silk, scoop neckline, sleeveless,
empire waistline, cummerbund, embroidery
appliqué, panel back, straight skirt.
$50-$75

Detail of appliqué

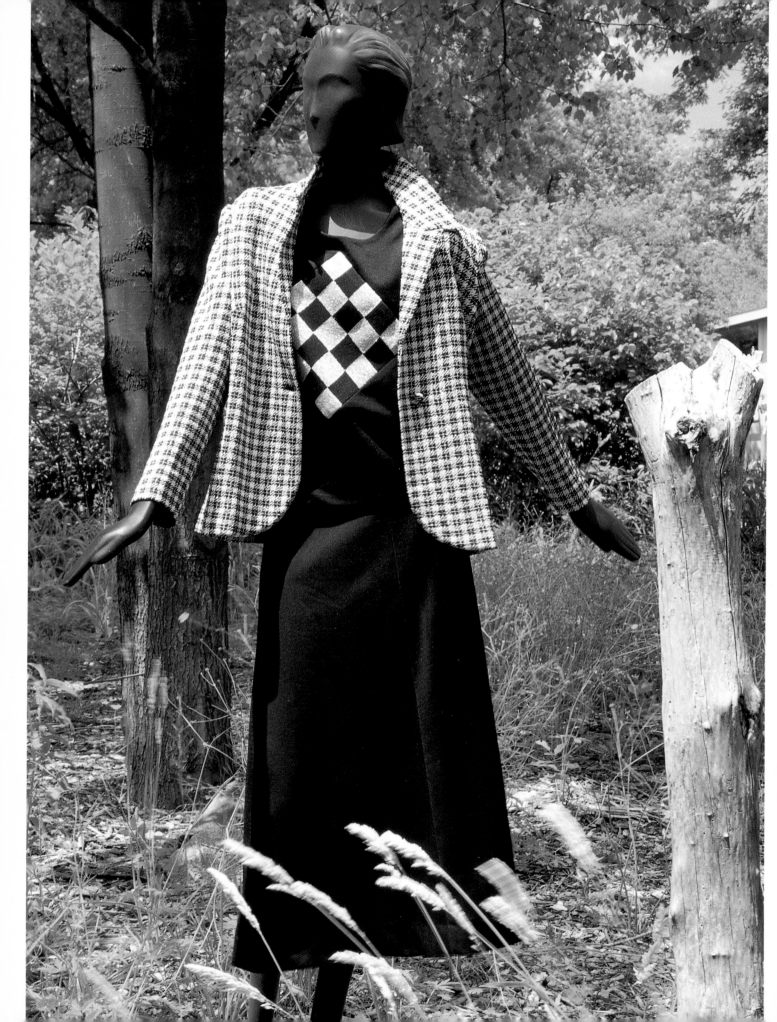

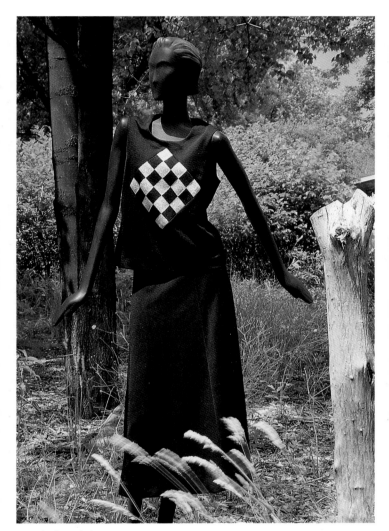

Shell and skirt

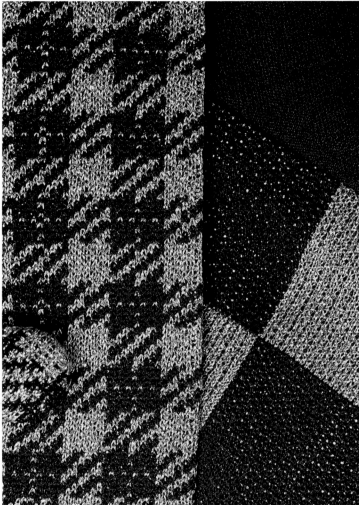

Detail of fabric

Opposite:
Evening Suit - c. 1970
Gino Paoli, Made in Italy
Black 100% polyester knit, silver lamé,
notched collar, shell with geometric
silver lamé panel, long slim skirt.
$100-$150

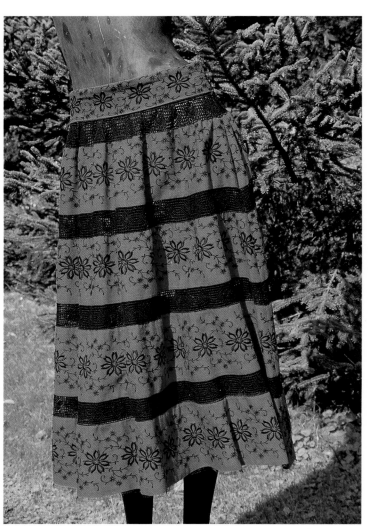

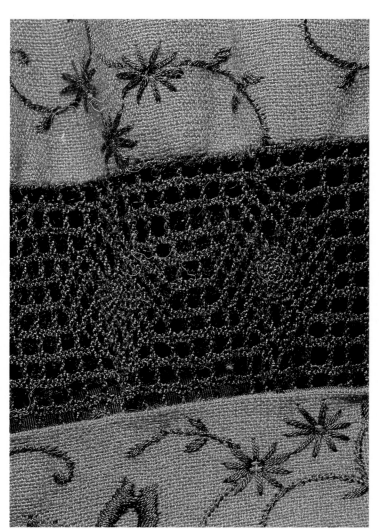

Evening skirt - c. 1960s
Melvine Miller
Rust 100% wool with black embroidery
and bands of black lace.
$175-$225
Courtesy Shirley Friedland

Detail of lace

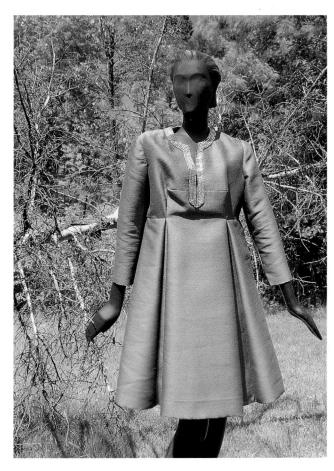

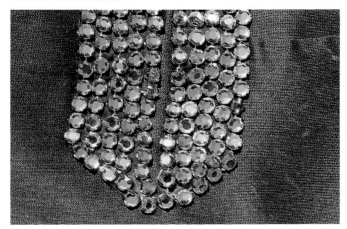

Left:
Evening dress - c. 1960s
Gunmetal grey 100% silk split round
neckline, long sleeve, rhinestone trim,
empire waistline, pleated skirt.
$100-$150

Below:
Detail of rhinestone trim

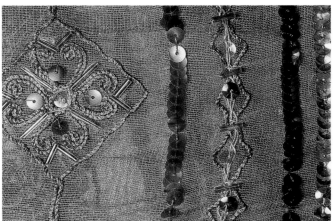

Right:
Evening dress - c. 1960s
Purple 100% silk, collar
tie, button closure, sequin
sleeve, gathered skirt.
$75-$125

Above:
Detail of trim

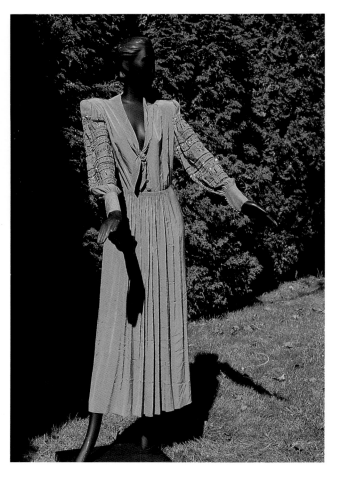

213

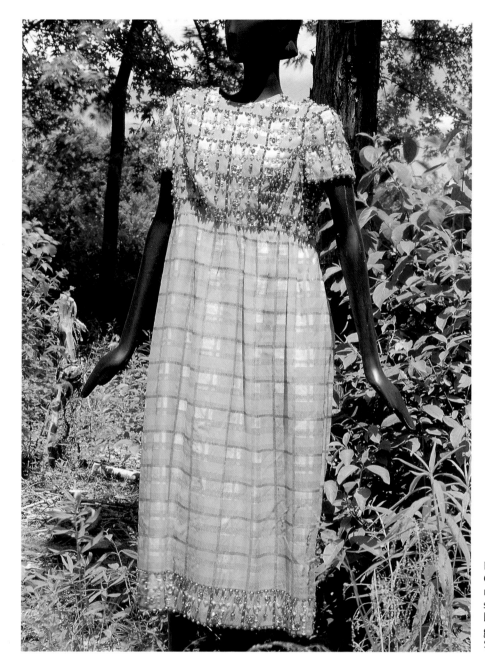

Evening dress - c. 1960s
Green 100% silk, plaid,
round neckline, short
sleeve, sequin crystal
beaded bodice,
gathered skirt.
$100-$150

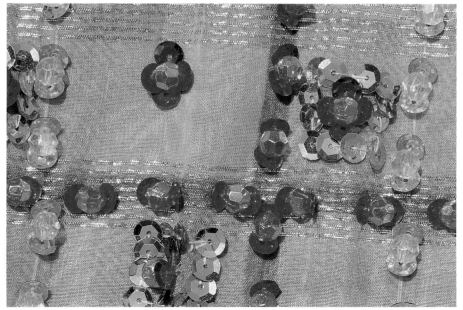

Detail of bead trim

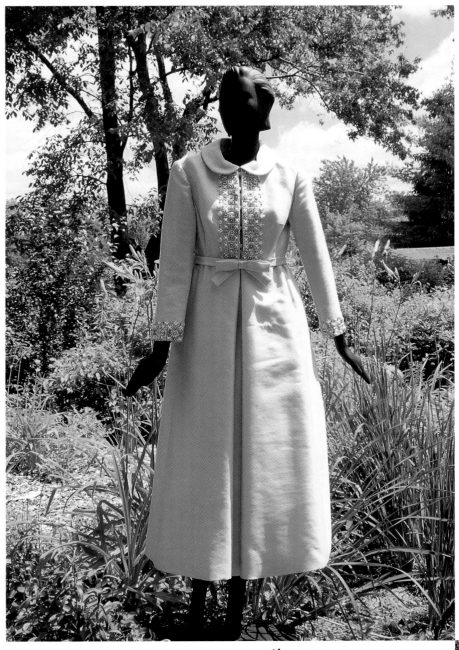

Above:
Evening gown - c. 1960s
Victoria Royal Ltd., Made in British
Crown Colony of Hong Kong
Pale green 100% silk, round collar,
long sleeve, gold rhinestone pearl
beaded bodice and cuff, bow
waistline, pleated skirt.
$150-$175

Right:
Detail of trim

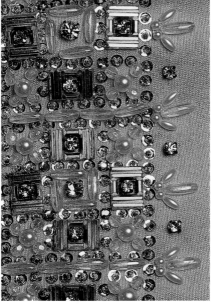

Evening gown - c. 1960s
Brown 100% rayon, round neckline, long
sleeve, empire waistline, gold braid trim.
$50-$75

Detail of braid

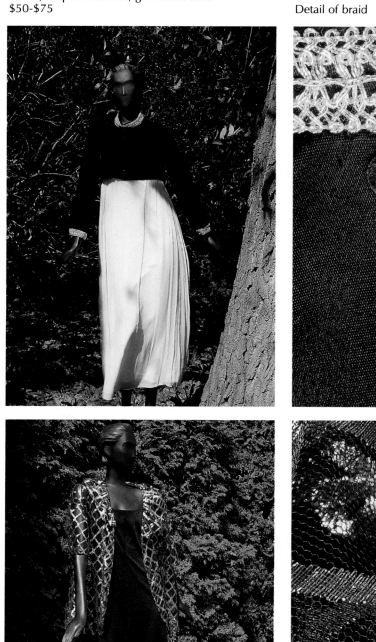

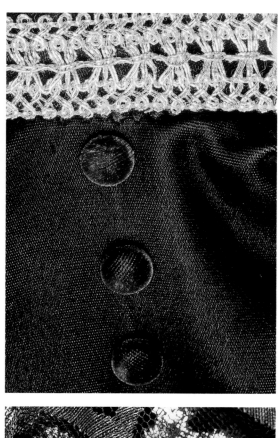

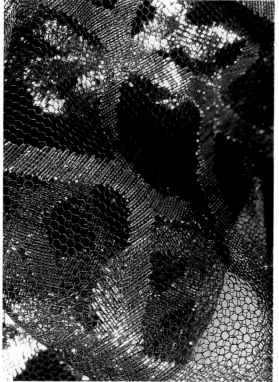

Evening gown - c. 1960s
Shady Lane, A Division of Jonathan Logan, Inc.
Black 100% polyester knit, scoop neckline,
sheath dress with silver lace jacket.
$100-125

Detail of lace

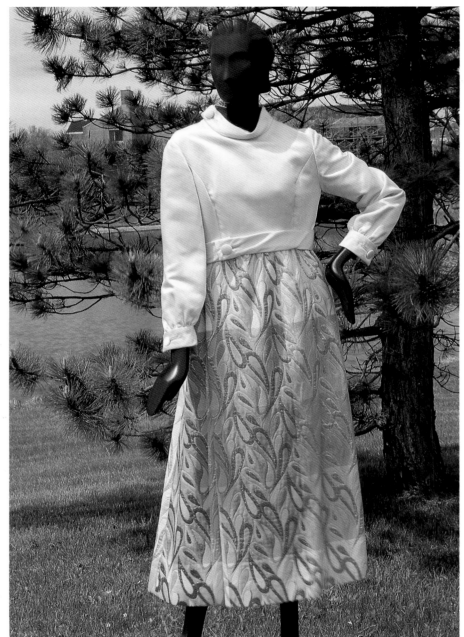

Evening gown - c. 1960s
Malcolm Starr International, Designed by
Rizkallah, Made in the
British Crown Colony of
Hong Kong
Yellow 100% silk, standing
collar, long sleeve,
brocade multi-color skirt.
$150-$200

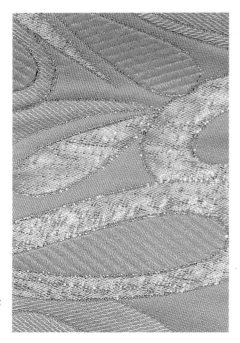

Detail of fabric

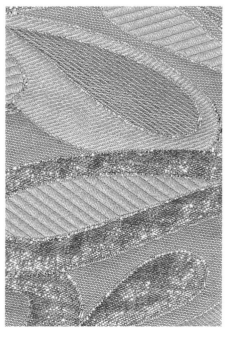

Detail of fabric

217

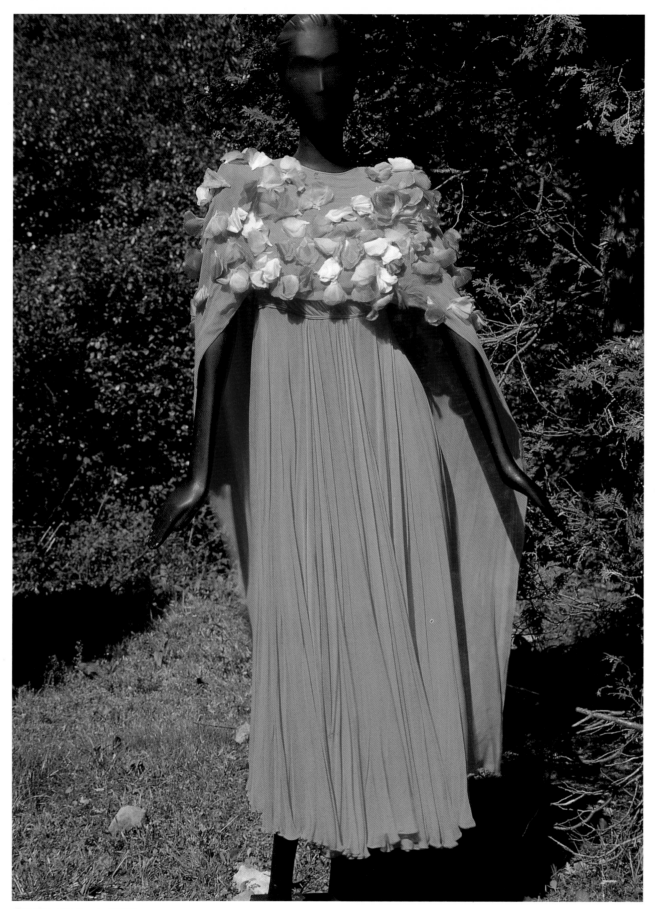

Evening gown - c. 1960s
Hot pink 100% silk chiffon, fitted bodice,
full skirt, long chiffon flower shawl.
$100-$150

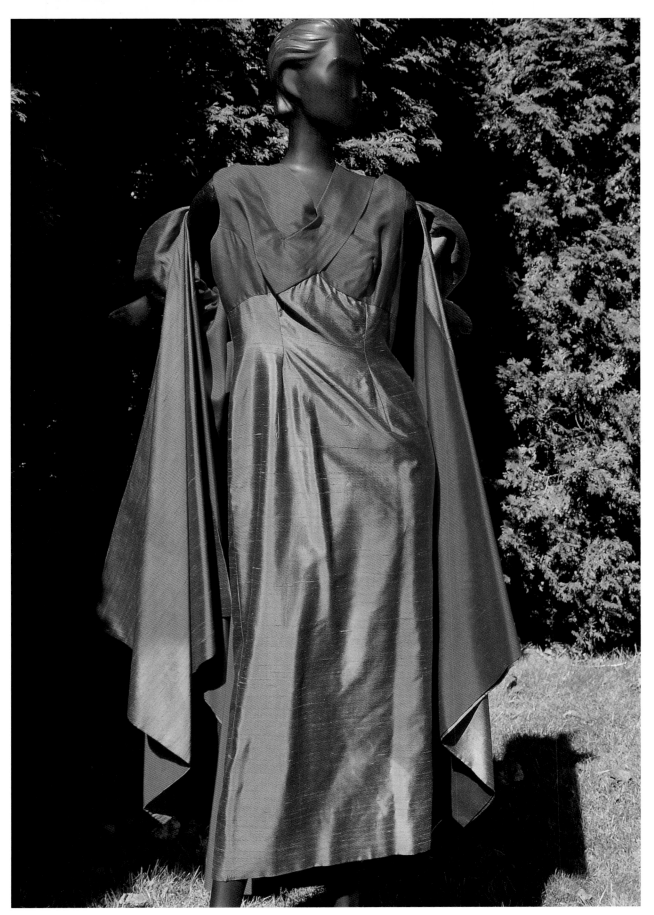

Evening gown - c. 1960s
Milgrim
Purple 100% silk, magenta bodice,
purple skirt, panel back, matching coat.
$150-$200

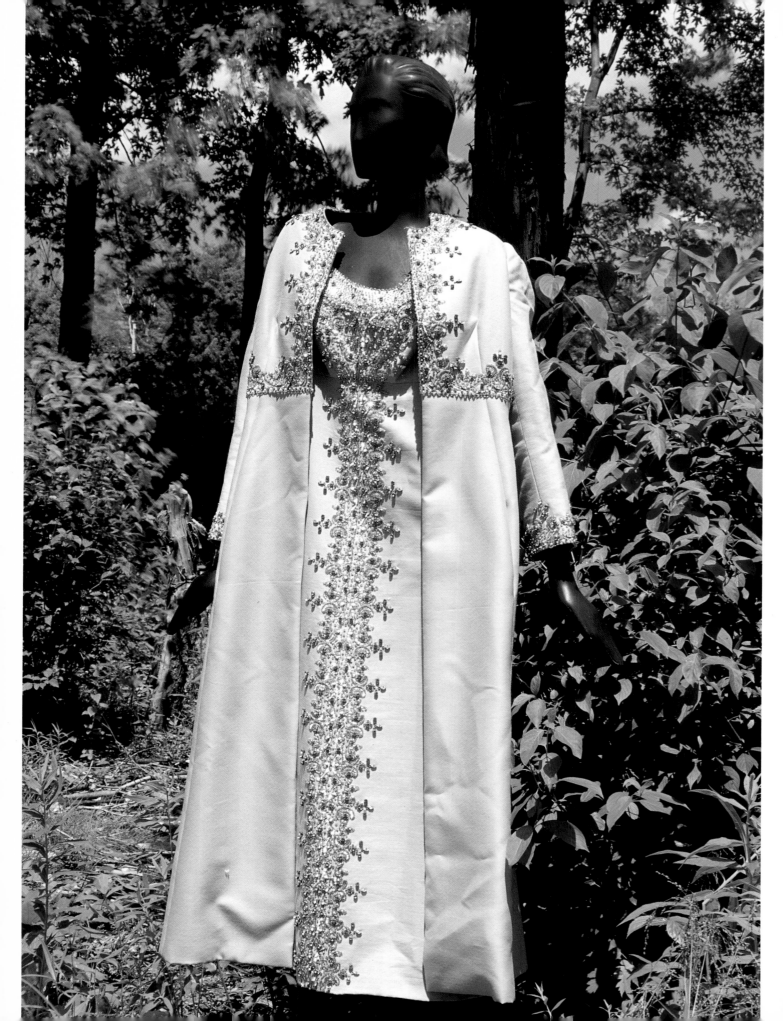

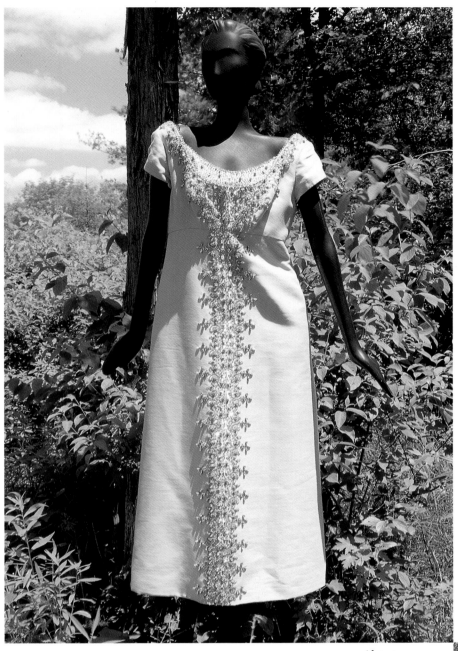

Above:
Dress

Right:
Detail of jewels

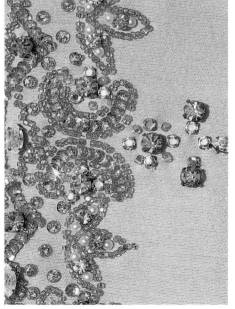

Opposite:
Evening Coat and Gown - c. 1960s
Seaton Enterprises Ltd., Made in British
Crown Colony of Hong Kong
Christian Dior knock-off, blue 100% silk,
evening coat, round neckline, long
sleeve, empire waist, jewel encrusted
bodice; evening dress, scoop neckline,
short sleeve, empire waist, jewel
encrusted bodice and front panel.
$250-$300

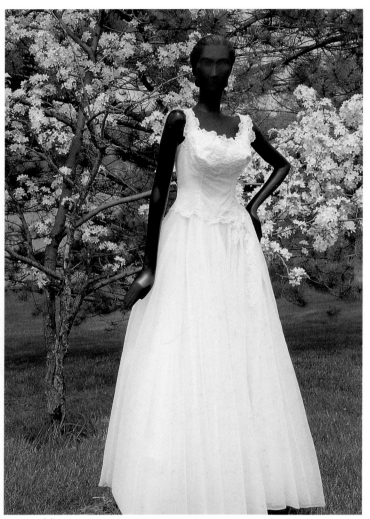

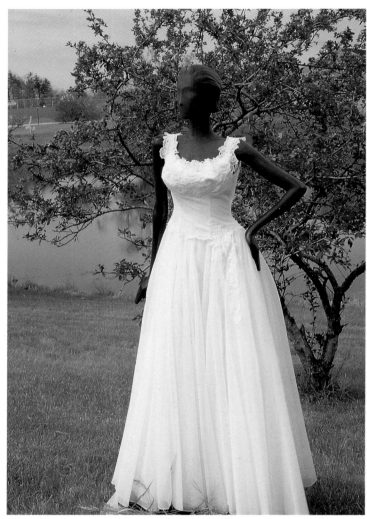

Wedding gown - c. 1959
White chiffon, fitted bodice
appliqué trim, scoop neckline,
sleeveless, full circle skirt.
$100-$150

Wedding gown - c. 1959
Different background

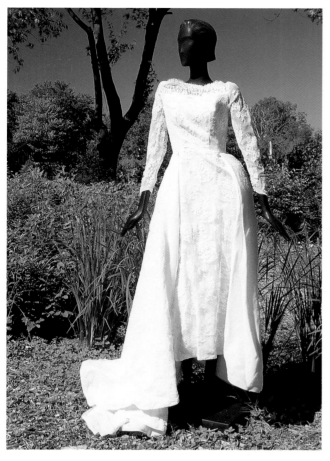

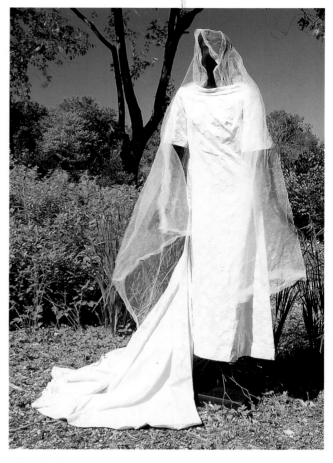

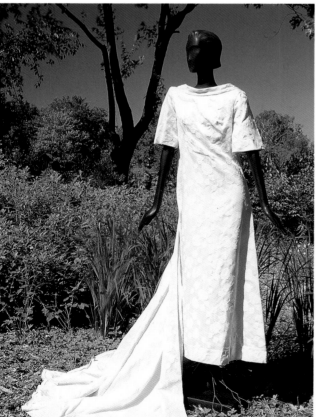

Above left:
Wedding gown - c. 1966
White 100% nylon, lace bodice,
scoop neckline, long sleeve,
sheath skirt, long train.
$100-$150
Author

Above right:
Wedding gown - c. 1967
Candlelight 100% silk brocade,
cowl collar neckline, 3/4 sleeve,
A-line silhouette, attached
shoulder train, cathedral length
veil.
$100-$150
Courtesy Barbara Johnson Cook

Left:
Wedding gown without
cathedral length veil.

Bibliography

Batterberry, Michael and Ariane. *Fashion The Mirror of History*. New York: Greenwich House, 1977.

Bond, David. *The Guinness Guide to 20th Century Fashion*. London: Guinness Superlatives Ltd., 1981.

Boucher, Francois. *20,000 Years of Fashion*. New York: Harry N. Abrams, Inc., 1967.

Calasibetta, Charlotte. *Essential Terms of Fashion: A Collection of Definitions*. New York: Fairchild Publications, Inc., 1985.

Calasibetta, Charlotte. *Fairchild's Dictionary of Fashion*. New York: Fairchild Publications, Inc., 1975.

Chase, Edna Woolman and Ilka Chase. *Always in Vogue*. New York: Doubleday & Company, Inc., 1954.

Coleridge, Nicholas. *The Fashion Conspiracy*. New York: Harper & Row, 1988.

Devlin, Polly. *Vogue Book of Fashion Photography*. New York: Simon and Schuster, 1979.

Dolan, Maryanne. *Vintage Clothing 1880-1960*. Florence, Alabama: Books Americana, 1987.

Dorner, J. *Fashion in the Forties and Fifties*. New Rochelle, New York: Arlington House Publishers, 1975.

Drake, Nicholas. *The Sixties: A Decade in Vogue*. Englewood Cliffs, New Jersey: Prentice-Hall, 1988.

Edelstein, Andrew J. *The Pop Sixties*. New York: World Almanac Publications, 1985.

Ewing, Elizabeth. *History of 20th Century Fashion*. New York: Charles Scribner's Sons, 1974.

Fogarty, Anne. *Wife-Dressing*. New York: Julian Messner Inc., 1959.

Gold, Annalee. *75 Years of Fashion*. New York: Fairchild Publications, 1975.

Horn, Marilyn J. *The Second Skin, An Interdisciplinary Study of Clothing*. New York: Houghton Mifflin Company, 1975.

Humphries, Mary. *Fabric Glossary*. Upper Saddle River, New Jersey: Prentice Hall, 1996.

Keenan, Brigid. *Dior in Vogue*. New York: Harmony Books, 1981.

Laver, James. *Costume and Fashion A Concise History*. London: Thames and Hudson Ltd., 1969.

Lobenthal, Joel. *Radical Rags Fashions of The Sixties*. New York: Abbeville Press, 1990.

Milbank, Carolyn. *New York Fashion: The Evolution of American Style*. New York: Harry N. Abrams, Inc., 1989.

Mulvagh, J. *Vogue History of 20th Century Fashion*. New York: Viking Penguin, 1988.

O'Hara, Georgina. *The Encyclopedia of Fashion*. New York: Harry N. Abrams, Inc., 1986.

Peacock, John. *Costume 1066-1966*. London: Thames and Hudson Ltd., 1986.

Ruby, Jennifer. *Costume in Context: 1940s and 1950s*. London: B. T. Batsford, 1987.

Ruby, Jennifer. *Costume in Context: 1960s and 1970s*. London: B. T. Batsford, 1989.

Schnurnberger, Lynn. *Let There by Clothes*. New York: Workman Publishing, 1991.

Stegemeyer, Anne. *Who's Who in Fashion*. New York: Fairchild Publications, 1980.

Tortora, Phyllis G. and Keith Eubank. *Survey of Historic Costume A History of Western Dress*. New York: Fairchild Publications, 1994.

Vogue Magazine. 1950-1970.

Timeline sources

Grun, Bernard. *The Timetables of History*. 3rd ed. New York: Simon & Schuster, 1991.

Hart, Michael H. *The 100: A Ranking of the Most Influential Persons in History*. New York: Hart Publications, 1978.

Hellemans, Alexander & Bryan Bunch. *The Timetables of Science*. New York: Simon & Schuster, 1988.

Layman, Richard, ed. *American Decades 1960-69*. Detroit: Gale Research, 1995.

Lee, Stan. *The Best of the World's Worst*. Los Angeles: General Publishing Group, 1994.

McFarland, Kevin. *Incredible People*. New York: Hart, 1975.

Panati, Charles. *Extraordinary Origins of Everyday Things*. New York: Harper & Row, 1987.

Smith, Godfrey ed. *1000 Makers of the Twentieth Century*. London: Times Newspapers, 1971.

Stewart, Robert. *Illustrated Almanac of Historical Facts*. New York: Prentice Hall, 1992.

Wallechinsky, Irvin, et al. *The Book of Lists*. New York: William Morrow, Co., 1977.